Handbook of Urologic Cryoablation

Handbook of Urologic Cryoablation

Edited by

Daniel B. Rukstalis MD
Director
Department of Urology
Geisinger Medical Center
Danville, PA
USA

Aaron Katz MD
Department of Urology
College of Physicians and Surgeons
Columbia University
New York, NY
USA

© 2007 Informa UK Ltd

First published in the United Kingdom in 2007 by Informa Healthcare, 4 Park Square, Milton Park, Abingdon, Oxon OX14 4RN. Informa Healthcare is a trading division of Informa UK Ltd. Registered Office: 37/41 Mortimer Street, London W1T 3JH. Registered in England and Wales number 1072954.

Tel: +44 (0)20 7017 6000
Fax: +44 (0)20 7017 6699
Email: info.medicine@tandf.co.uk
Website: www.tandf.co.uk/medicine

A CIP record for this book is available from the British Library.

Library of Congress Cataloging-in-Publication Data
Data available on application

ISBN-10: 1 84184 577 9
ISBN-13: 978 1 84184 577 7

Distributed in North and South America by
Taylor & Francis
6000 Broken Sound Parkway, NW, (Suite 300)
Boca Raton, FL 33487, USA

Within Continental USA
Tel: 1 (800) 272 7737; Fax: 1 (800) 374 3401
Outside Continental USA
Tel: (561) 994 0555; Fax: (561) 361 6018
Email: orders@crcpress.com

Distributed in the rest of the world by
Thomson Publishing Services
Cheriton House
North Way
Andover, Hampshire SP10 5BE, UK
Tel: +44 (0)1264 332424
Email: tps.tandfsalesorder@thomson.com

Composition by Exeter Premedia Services Private Ltd., Chennai, India
Printed and bound in India by Replika Press Pvt Ltd

Contents

Contributors

John G. Baust
Department of Biological Sciences
State University of New York
Binghamton, NY
USA

John M. Baust
Department of Biological Sciences
State University of New York
Binghamton, NY
USA

Arie S. Belldegrun MD
Department of Urology
David Geffen School of Medicine at UCLA
Los Angeles, CA
USA

David G. Bostwick MD
Bostwick Laboratories
Glen Allen, VA
USA

Ralph V. Clayman MD
Department of Urology
University of California
Irvine, CA
USA

Jeffrey K. Cohen
Triangle Urology
Pittsburgh, PA
USA

Sean M. Collins MD
Department of Urology
College of Physicians and Surgeons
Columbia University
New York, NY
USA

John Danella
Geisinger Health System
Division of Urology
Danville, PA
USA

Patrick Davol
Geisinger Health System
Division of Urology
Danville, PA
USA

Leslie A. Deane MB BS
Department of Urology
University of California
Irvine, CA
USA

Michael Enriquez MHA, CHE
Division of Surgery
Geisinger Health System
Danville, PA
USA

Brant R. Fulmer MD
Associate in Urology
Geisinger Health System
Danville, PA
USA

Andrew A. Gage
Department of Surgery
State University of New York
Buffalo, NY
USA

Daniel Hendricks CPA
Division of Surgery
Geisinger Health System
Danville, PA
USA

Aaron Katz MD
Department of Urology
College of Physicians and Surgeons
Columbia University
New York, NY
USA

Kristin Kozakowski MD
Department of Urology
College of Physicians and Surgeons
Columbia University
New York, NY
USA

John S. Lam MD
Department of Urology
David Geffen School of Medicine at UCLA
Los Angeles, CA
USA

Michael J. Manyak MD FACS
Department of Urology
The George Washington University Medical Center
Washington DC
USA

Isabelle Meiers MD
Bostwick Laboratories
Glen Allen, VA
USA

Ralph J. Miller Jr MD
Triangle Urology
Pittsburgh, PA
USA

Michelle Nagel CPC
Professional Reimbursement and Compliance
Geisinger Health System
Danville, PA
USA

Stephen Y. Nakada MD
Division of Urology, Department of Surgery
University of Wisconsin-Madison Medical School
Madison, WI
USA

Daniel B. Rukstalis MD
Director
Department of Urology
Geisinger Medical Center
Danville, PA
USA

Peter G. Schulam MD PhD
Department of Urology
David Geffen School of Medicine at UCLA
Los Angeles, CA
USA

W. Bruce Shingleton MD
Department of Urology
Louisiana State University Health Science Center
Shreveport, LA
USA

Jennifer Simmons MD
Geisinger Health System
Division of Urology
Danville, PA
USA

Charles Wen MD
Division of Urology, Department of Surgery
University of Wisconsin-Madison Medical School
Madison, WI
USA

Foreword

Due to advances in abdominal imaging over the past 30 years, there has been a notable increase in incidentally discovered small renal tumors, many of which have questionable malignant potential. Likewise, the discovery and use of PSA for prostate cancer screening has led to a phase shift in prostate cancer detection, allowing more men to undergo curative treatment for early, localized prostate cancer. As many of these patients are asymptomatic when faced with this situation, they will educate themselves on traditional treatments as well as occasionally seeking out less invasive therapies. Cryoablation, radiofrequency ablation (RFA) and high-intensity frequency ultrasound (HIFU) are considered possible alternatives to the time-honored extirpative procedures of radical (or partial) nephrectomy and radical retropubic prostatectomy (RRP). Although early in their evolution, these alternatives have the potential to fit the ideal definition of an effective minimally invasive oncologic therapy; that is, one that completely ablates cancerous tissue yet spares patients the morbidity often experienced following traditional treatments. Open and laparoscopic prostatectomy involves a major anatomic disruption and even in the most experienced hands can result in significant patient morbidity. The most common morbidities of urinary incontinence and impotence have been reduced by continued improvements in technique. In fact, continence rates in excess of 90% and potency rates greater than 70% are now routinely observed in high-volume centers following either open or laparoscopic radical prostatectomy. However, attaining these results takes many years of training, hundreds to thousands of cases, and a career dedicated to further refinement in technique. In regards to minimizing the morbidity of renal and prostate surgery, cryoablation is perhaps the most thoroughly studied of the minimally invasive ablative therapies.

Cryoablation or cryosurgery is defined as the use of freezing to destroy or excise tissue. The use of subfreezing temperatures to ablate tissue has a long history in medicine dating back to 19th century England. The process was referred to as congelation (the process of congealing or solidification) and was first used and described by James Arnott in 1850.[1] He applied a frigorific mixture consisting of pounded ice and various salts to the perineum of a 42-year-old woman with ulcerative uterine cancer. After at least 30 applications he described excitedly that "no advance of the disease appears ... and in other respects there is decided improvement ... she is stronger and able to occupy herself in the usual household affairs." Arnott was obviously years ahead of his time and surmised that the application of cold could not only be used for palliation but could potentially treat cancer, "Whether more is to be expected from it – whether, in the early stages especially, it may not possess energies equal to the complete removal of the disease – is a point that must be decided by further experience." Following Arnott's experience, the use of cold continued through the turn of the century as liquefied gases became available. Liquefied air (−190°C), oxygen (−182.9°C) and solid carbon dioxide (−78.5°C) were applied topically to treat dermatologic lesions.[2] It was in the mid 20th century that Cooper, a neurosurgeon, ushered in the modern era of cryoablation by using a liquid nitrogen probe to perform stereotactic cryoablation of the basal ganglion.[3] His liquid nitrogen apparatus was analogous to many modern cryoablative systems in that all but the tip of the probe was insulated and a thermocouple measured distal probe temperature. Cooper successfully treated thousands of patients with tremors and involuntary movements characteristic of Parkinsonism until the advent of L-dopa in the late 1960s. The 1960s also produced the first studies in which renal and prostate tissue were specifically targeted. Moreover, the field of cryoimmunology was born when researchers were able to induce circulating antibodies against antigens from the frozen tissue of rabbit seminal vesicles.[4]

These studies form the foundation of today's practice of cryoablation. Kidney tumors are an especially attractive target as the iceball can be readily monitored during freezing using ultrasound. Moreover, patients can undergo periodic follow-up imaging either with CT or MRI. Tumors have been ablated after open or laparoscopic mobilization of the kidney, and percutaneously using ultrasound, CT, or MRI guidance. Enhancement following intravenous contrast administration is currently our best surrogate for recurrence or treatment failure. In the future we may need to rely more heavily on functional imaging modalities such as PET or a combination of PET and CT.

Prospective surveillance of patients following renal tumor ablation has been limited to a handful of larger centers. Currently, most procedures are, quite appropriately, performed on patients who are elderly or are poor operative candidates. The Cleveland Clinic has provided us with 3 years of follow-up data detailing the success of laparoscopic cryoablation in selected patients. Although extremely promising as an ablative modality, we will need 10-year follow-up data showing equivalence to traditional nephrectomy or partial nephrectomy before we can safely broaden the indications to include younger, healthier patients.

In the future, the majority of renal tumors treated with cryoablation will probably be dealt with percutaneously. Currently, posterior, exophytic tumors are especially well suited for this approach, as patients require only local anesthesia with little or no sedation. Most groups administer the treatment with the aid of CT or MRI guidance, taking advantage of their excellent spatial resolution, although ultrasound guidance can also be used. Ultimately the success of a particular ablative therapy, be it RFA or cryoablation, is probably most dependent on technique and less on the actual energy modality applied. As a result, cooperation between urologist and radiologist is paramount to the successful treatment of these lesions. Each specialist brings to the table a unique perspective and the patients ultimately benefit from a cooperative union of these experiences. The success of this approach likely lies with a symbiotic relationship between the two specialties.

In 1964, Gonder et al ushered in the era of prostate cryotherapy by applying liquid nitrogen probes to the dog prostate. They were able to demonstrate postoperative necrosis, resorption, and decreased prostate size.[5] Unlike renal tumor procedures, prostate cancer treatments are judged not only on oncologic efficacy but also on their effect on continence and sexual function. Throughout the 1970s and into the 1980s, cryoablation for prostate cancer was fraught with complications because of a lack of precision during the freezing phase. In the 1990s there was resurgence in prostatic cryoablation mainly due to the development of smaller probes and improved ultrasonic monitoring of the cryolesion. Urethral warming catheters were also used to reduce the incidence of sloughing and stricture formation. Despite these improvements, impotence remained the rule rather than the exception following prostatic cryoablation.

Prostate cryoablation has been used as salvage therapy for recurrence after brachytherapy or external beam radiation (EBR). Although the risk of incontinence after salvage cryoablation is lower than after RRP, more prospective trials will be needed to show oncologic results equivalent to salvage RRP. Recent trials have used primary cryoablation for localized prostate cancer. Currently, we lack evidence that this modality is as effective as traditional therapies of EBR, RRP or brachytherapy. Moreover, nerve-sparing cryoablation is in its infancy and is probably warranted only in controlled trial settings. Nevertheless, prostatic cryoablation technology continues to evolve.

Rectourethral fistula formation, once fairly common, is exceedingly rare in contemporary series. The risk of incontinence is now comparable to RRP in experienced hands. Therefore, although impotence is common following cryoablation, it may be a viable alternative in men in whom sexual function is not a priority or who are already impotent.

In conclusion, cryoablation is a promising modality, which has been proven to exhibit complete tumor cell kill to a specified area of tissue. This text provides the reader with a comprehensive understanding of the science and clinical application of cryoablation with respect to urology. We have come a long way from Arnott's congelation in 1850 and this exciting technology is certainly here to stay. It would be wise for all urologists to become familiar with the fundamentals of cryobiology as well as have a basic understanding of the application of cryotherapy in renal and prostate tumors. It is furthermore paramount that urologists apply these new technologies in carefully controlled settings. Too often new technologies are applied in uncontrolled settings at the behest of industry. In view of that, it should remain for us as physicians to determine and develop the best treatments for our patients. With further refinement, and prospective, multi-institutional trials, we will ultimately realize the full potential of cryoablation.

Andrew A. Wagner and Alan W. Partin

REFERENCES

1. Arnott J. Practical illustrations of the remedial efficacy of a very low or anaesthetic temperature. I. in cancer. Lancet 1850; 2: 257–318.
2. Gage AA. History of cryosurgery. Semin Surg Oncol 1998; 14(2): 99–109.
3. Cooper IS. Cryogenic surgery: a new method of destruction or extirpation of benign or malignant tissues. N Engl J Med 1963; 268: 743–9.
4. Yantorno C, Soanes WA, Gonder MJ, Shulman S. Studies in cryoimmunology. I. The production of antibodies to urogenital tissue in consequence of freezing treatment. Immunology 1967; 12(4): 395–410.
5. Gonder MJ, Soanes WA, Smith V. Experimental prostate cryosurgery. Invest Urol 1964; 14: 610–19.

Preface

Humankind, from the early Neanderthals to the passengers and crew of the Titanic, has long understood one fact; cold temperatures kill. However, it wasn't until the 1950s that the lethal power of cold could be harnessed and directed against specific human diseases such as cancer. Initially, liquid nitrogen was pumped through metal needles that had been placed under visual guidance into a specific disease site. The early cryosurgeon then used visual cues and an intrinsic understanding of three-dimensional anatomy to control the extent of the cold-induced injury. Predictably, the targeted tissue was indeed killed. However, the adjacent, and often vital, structures were also injured with many adverse outcomes.

Technical improvements in the delivery of cold-inducing cryogens such as liquid nitrogen and high-pressure argon gas in the 1990s rejuvenated the *in situ* ablative treatment approach. The final tipping point was reached when body imaging modalities such as ultrasound (US), computed tomography (CT), and magnetic resonance (MRI) were used to directly monitor the location and extent of the ablation zone. The ice created by the cryo-units was found to be hyperechoic on ultrasound and easily visible on both CT and MRI. Finally, the concept of image-guided tissue ablation was successfully extended beyond the boundaries of radiation therapy. Currently, individuals who find themselves in the complex circumstance of harboring a cancer within an organ or tissue that is closely approximated to other vital structures can choose from an array of ablative techniques that can be individualized to their specific illness.

The development of special equipment for the thermal destruction, with both cold injury and heat induced tissue necrosis, of neoplastic lesions within the adrenal gland, kidney and prostate has contributed to the recent establishment of the new medical specialty of interventional oncology. The wide availability of the required equipment has allowed individual medical practitioners from urology, surgical oncology, thoracic surgery and interventional radiology to treat cancers that were previously only treated with surgical excision or radiation therapy. These new treatment options hold much promise for the effective treatment of early cancers while reducing the treatment-related side effects associated with more traditional modalities. However, these new treatment approaches also serve to break down the well-established distinctions between medical specialties, which can result in confusion, and tension between those specialties. Until the various physicians can develop new systems of communication that deliver medical care as a team-based treatment unit, patients may find themselves receiving conflicting opinions about the optimal therapy for their specific problem. Finally, the usual method through which physicians evaluate new treatment strategies over time is being taxed by the rapid identification of ever more effective inventions for tissue ablation. Concomitantly, payment mechanisms must be continually adjusted such that men and women with cancer can receive the benefit of these attractive new modalities.

This *"Handbook of Urologic Cryoablation"* has been developed to present the current best evidence in the field of tissue ablation and interventional oncology as it applies to the field of urologic oncology. The authors who have contributed chapters for this book are experienced with the engineering of the specific equipment, its history of development and the rationale for its application in the treatment of urologic disease.

Additionally, information has been provided regarding the economics of an ablation program such that interested readers can establish a clinical program that will enable them to readily apply this new knowledge to their patients.

Daniel B. Rukstalis and Aaron Katz

Acknowledgments

This book represents the collective contributions of all the innovators, engineers, physicians, hospital finance departments and support staff that have labored to give birth to the ablation industry over the past 15 years.

Color Plates

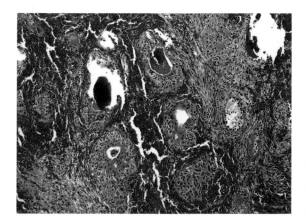

Figure 3.1 Stromal hemorrhage with residual viable epithelium following prostatic cryoablation (×100 magnification).

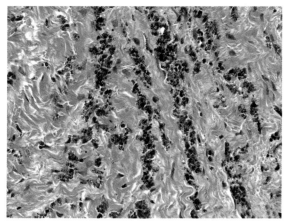

Figure 3.2 Hemosiderin deposition (ochre pigment) within the stroma after cryosurgery (×400 magnification).

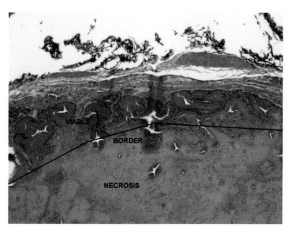

Figure 3.3 Coagulative necrosis (bottom of image) with devitalization and a thin rim of subcapsular viable tissue (top) following cryosurgery; dog prostate (×100 magnification).

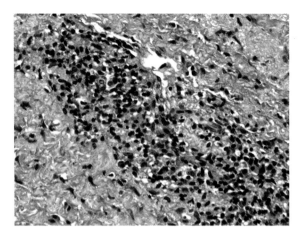

Figure 3.4 Patchy chronic inflammation within prostatic stroma is a common finding following cryoablation (×400 magnification).

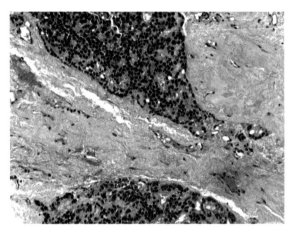

Figure 3.5 Residual/ recurrent adenocarcinoma (Gleason 4 + 4 = 8) indicating lack of treatment effect; tumor appeared unchanged, with no change in grade or definite evidence of tissue or immune response (×200 magnification).

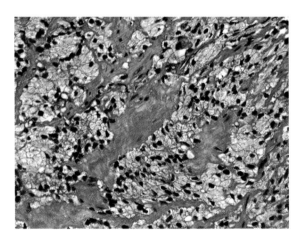

Figure 3.6A Residual/ recurrent adenocarcinoma (Gleason 4 + 3 = 7) (400× magnification).

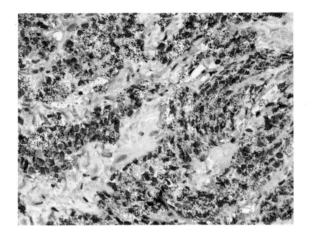

Figure 3.6B Intense racemase stain in cancer. There is prominent immunoreactivity (granular red reaction product) in most of the secretory cells. There is no immunoreactivity (absence of brown reaction product) for basal cell-specific high-molecular-weight keratin (34βE12) and p63 (400× magnification).

Visualizing renal cryoablation

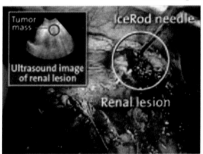

1. Identify the lesion

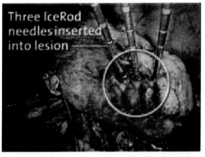

2. Cryoablation needles placed inside the lesion

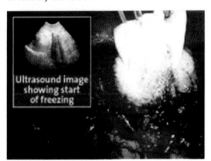

3. Monitoring iceball growth with real-time ultrasound guidance

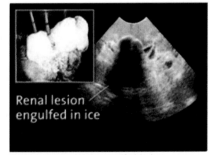

4. Lesion completely engulfed in ice

Figure 8.5 Step-by-step illustration of laparoscopic renal cryoablation with ultrasound correlation (courtesy of Oncura, Inc., Plymouth Meeting, PA).

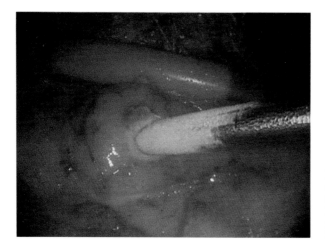

Figure 11.3 Laparoscopic-assisted cryoablation of an exophytic renal lesion. Laparoscopic ultrasound probe behind the lesion monitors the iceball growth.

1

Principles of cryosurgical technique

Andrew A. Gage, John M. Baust, John G. Baust

Introduction • **The mechanisms of injury** • **The freeze–thaw cycle** • **Implications for clinical technique** • **Summary**

INTRODUCTION

Cryosurgery requires the removal of heat from the tissues, thereby producing localized freezing to an appropriate extent for therapy. The procedure is based on established well-known cryobiological principles, which originally were formed during investigative work on cryopreservation of cells and tissues and on the pathogenesis of frostbite. From the beginning of the modern era of cryosurgery, when automated cryosurgical equipment became available early in the 1960s, dosimetry in terms of temperature and duration of the freeze–thaw cycle was an important issue. In the 1960s, Cooper wrote that a tissue temperature of $-20°C$ or colder, held for 1 minute or longer, was sufficient to produce necrosis of tissue.[1,2] This statement was based on his experimental work but also has some basis on investigations of frostbite.[3] Nevertheless it soon became evident that this elevated freezing temperature was not adequate for the treatment of tumors. In the following years, experimental investigations and clinical reports have attempted to define the appropriate temperature–time dosimetry of cryosurgery for tissue ablation. A diversity of opinions and practices, caused by the variability in thermal gradients in frozen tissue, blood flow, anatomy, accessory warmers, etc., has become evident, so dosimetry remains a matter of concern. This chapter defines the optimal technique for urological cryosurgery, including recognition of the anatomical constraints, and provides a view of the adjunctive therapy needed to increase the efficacy of cryosurgery for tumors of the kidney and prostate gland.

THE MECHANISMS OF INJURY

Cryosurgical treatment requires that a volume of tissue be frozen, using appropriate techniques and instruments to monitor and control the freezing process. When used for tumors, the intent is to produce destruction of the neoplasm, so the need for precision in treatment is substantial. An understanding of the mechanisms of injury is essential for efficacious treatment.

The destructive effects of freezing tissue, as practiced in cryosurgical treatment, are due to a number of factors which may be divided into two major mechanisms: immediate and delayed injury. The immediate cause of injury is the deleterious effect of freezing and thawing on the cells. The delayed cause of injury follows thawing when microcirculatory failure and vascular stasis develop. The relative importance of these two mechanisms of injury has long been debated in explanations of the pathogenesis of frostbite injury and that debate continues in recent investigations on the nature of injury in cryosurgery. Research on this subject is complicated by the dual nature of injury. Research *in vitro* provides an understanding of the direct deleterious effects of freezing on cells and tissues, but cannot take into account the effect of changes in blood flow. Research *in vivo* must evaluate a complex injury. Varying thermal conditions in the frozen volume of tissue are present. Repetitive freeze–thaw cycles further disturb the focus on any one phase of the freeze–thaw cycle. Then the development of vascular stasis and tissue ischemia obscures the effect of freezing caused by direct cell injury. Nevertheless, clearly, both mechanisms of injury are operative in cryosurgery and merit understanding for precision in this therapeutic modality.

The deleterious effects of low temperature on cells begins early in hypothermia. As the temperature falls, the structure and function of cells, including their constituent proteins and lipids are stressed. Cell metabolism progressively fails (uncouples) as temperature falls, and death may follow even though the cell was not subjected to freezing temperatures. In cryosurgery, hypothermia, an initiating stress, is present for many minutes before and after the procedure, including in the tissue immediately surrounding the frozen volume.

As the temperature falls into the freezing range, water is crystallized and "removed" as a biologically functional compound. Ice crystal formation is a cornerstone of cryogenic injury and may occur both in extracellular spaces and within the cell, depending upon the rapidity and duration of cooling. Slow cooling, that is, 10°C/minute or less, will produce ice crystal formation in the extracellular spaces, creating a hyperosmotic extracellular environment, which in turn draws water from the cells yielding final osmolalities of 8–10 osm. The cells are diminished in size and membranes, cellular constituents are damaged, and cell death may result. The deleterious effects of cell dehydration and increased solute concentration are collectively known as solute effects injury. With further cooling, ice crystals may form within the cells. Many cells may contain ice crystals by −15°C (heterogeneous nucleation). The manner in which extracellular ice crystals enter a cell is uncertain. Perhaps the increased osmotic pressure produced by ice crystal formation damages the cell membrane to an extent that permits penetration by ice crystals. As an alternative, ice crystals may enter the cell through micropores in the membrane.[4,5] The extracellular ice formation, which contributes to the solute effects, is not necessarily lethal for cells. However, intracellular ice damages the cell membrane and organelles and is considered lethal, though some exceptions are cited by Mazur.[6] Probabilistic certainty of intracellular ice formation requires temperatures colder than −40°C (homogeneous nucleation).[7] Rapid cooling rates, that is, 100°C/minute and greater, will produce intracellular ice crystals because the water will not have adequate time needed to leave the cell.

The propagation of ice crystals during the freezing of tissue has been shown to extend through the lumen of blood vessels or ductal structures, which provide channels of decreased resistance.[8,9] Experiments with breast tissue demonstrated that ice formed in the connective tissue and propagated through the connective tissue.[10] Experiments *in vitro* with salivary glands have demonstrated cell-to-cell propagation via intercellular channels.[11] The masses of frozen cells, closely packed as tissue in clinical applications of cryosurgery, are subjected to the shearing forces of ice crystal formation and this mechanical effect will disrupt the tissue structure and have deleterious effects, regardless of whether the ice crystals are extracellular or intracellular. During thawing, ice crystals grow in size, fusing to form large crystals. This process, called recrystallization, occurs most noticeably at temperatures in the range of −20 to −40°C. In tissues with closely packed cells, the mechanical forces produced by the large crystals are disruptive and increase the chance of cell death.

Microcirculatory failure, producing vascular stasis, is a major mechanism of cell death in cryosurgery. The sequence of events is well demonstrated in experiments on the pathogenesis of frostbite and in cryosurgical investigations in a variety of tissues. The sequence of events after freezing and thawing has been observed in thin transilluminated tissues, including the mesentery and the cheek pouches of hamsters.[12-14] Experiments with diverse tissues, such as the rat liver, hamster cheek pouch, and guinea pig skin, have shown that vascular changes occur at temperatures as warm as −20°C.[15-24] The initial response to the cooling of tissues is vasoconstriction and a reduction in blood flow. When the tissue is frozen, circulation ceases. When the tissue thaws, circulation is briefly restored, at first showing a degree of hyperemia because of vasodilation. Damage to the endothelial cells results in increased permeability of the capillary walls, leading to platelet aggregation and microthrombus formation in the initial hour or two after thawing.[25-28] Edema develops in this time. Many small blood vessels are occluded by 4 hours after thawing, but arterioles may remain patent for 24 hours. The loss of blood supply results in complete cell death in the ischemic tissue, except at the periphery of the previously frozen volume of tissue.

The vascular response to freezing and the complete necrosis in the central cryogenic lesion have convinced many investigators that the main mechanism of cell death in cryosurgery is ischemia.[3,19,29] Efforts have been made to study the comparative effects of direct cell injury versus vascular stasis, as causes of tissue injury. Investigations supporting the importance of vascular injury note that tumor tissues excised immediately after a freeze–thaw cycle were transplanted successfully, but tumor tissue excised 48 hours after freezing–thawing did not survive transplantation.[30] These studies revealed that a number of alterations take place in tissues following cryoablation contributing to continued cell death in a delayed manner. Historically this delayed and extended cell death period was believed to be strictly a result of hypoxic and ischemic injury as discussed earlier. Recently a number of reports have demonstrated that much of the delayed cell death associated with cryoablation is a result of induction of the apoptotic cell death mechanisms.[31] In 1998, Baust et al first demonstrated that, following a freezing insult (cryopreservation), there was an activation of cell signaling cascades resulting in apoptosis. Further studies into freezing-induced cell death revealed that there was a temporal component to the manifestation of total molecular cell death following a freeze insult.[32] This temporal component has been termed "delayed-onset cell death" (DOCD). DOCD encompasses the entirety of cell death following a freeze insult in which a molecular response within a cell results in cell death. These events, including apoptosis, delayed necrosis, and secondary necrosis, contribute to much of the delayed cell death originally classified as ischemic injury and vascular necrosis. While difficult to differentiate solely with *in vivo* studies, modern molecular *in vitro* analysis has allowed for the characterization of the contribution and extent of the delayed-onset cell death, revealing a significant contribution.[31] Nevertheless, direct cell injury is an important mechanism of cell death, so careful attention must be given to all phases of the freeze–thaw cycle to maximize efficacy of cryosurgery.

THE FREEZE–THAW CYCLE

The knowledge critical to cryosurgical technique is related to the freeze–thaw cycle and its component phases. The precise details of experiments or clinical applications are difficult to describe because variances in the cooling–warming parameters and thermal profiles exist in the diverse regions of the frozen volume of tissue. For example, the tissue close to a cryosurgical probe cools rapidly while the tissue in a peripheral location cools slowly. The coldest temperatures reached and the time required for thawing vary, depending on the distance from the probe. Therefore the experimental or clinical application is described commonly in terms of the coldest temperature reached or in terms of the volume of tissue frozen. Sometimes only the probe temperature is reported, but this is of limited value. Cryosurgical research has shown that any part of the freeze–thaw cycle, such as the cooling rate, temperature produced in the tissue, and warming rate may be injurious. Therefore, knowledge of the effect of each phase of the freeze–thaw cycle is important.

The cooling rate ideally should be as rapid as possible because a fast cooling rate is likely to produce the lethal intracellular ice crystals. However, cryobiological studies have shown that a wide range of cooling rates may be associated with the formation of intracellular ice crystals. For examples, the following experiments are cited. In experiments with Dunning AT-1 tumor cells, the cooling rate needed to produce intracellular ice was 50°C/minute.[33] In experiments with slices of liver, intracellular ice crystals were seen at a cooling rate of 22°C/minute.[9] In neoplastic cells, frozen *in vitro* as tissue slices, intracellular ice crystals were observed at a cooling rate as slow as 3°C/minute, which was attributed to the possibility that tightly packed neoplastic cells might be more resistant to dehydration than cells in suspension.[34] In cell suspensions, cooling rates as low as 1°C/minute may produce intracellular ice.[6] Nevertheless such slow cooling rates are not likely to form a volume of intracellular ice crystals adequate to ensure complete ablation of the targeted tissue mass. Cellular dehydration that accompanies slow cooling may well serve a protective role.

In cryosurgical techniques, rapid tissue cooling, that is, of the order of 50°C/minute, is produced only very close to the cryosurgical probe. The further away from the probe, the slower is the tissue cooling rate, so that the cooling rate may be only 10 to 20°C/minute at a distance of 1 cm from the probe.[32] At a greater distance, the cooling rate will be very slow, so a significant amount of intracellular ice is unlikely. Freeze-substitution techniques have shown that intracellular ice crystals occur near the cryosurgical probe where the tissue cooling rate is high and that extracellular ice crystals and shrunken cells are seen at the periphery of the frozen volume where the cooling rate is slow.[35] In the cryosurgical treatment of tumors, most of the frozen volumes of tissues are not subjected to fast cooling rates. Therefore, slow cooling rates do not appear to be of primary importance in direct tissue injury from freezing, a view supported by Mazur and by Farrant and Walter.[6,36]

The treatment of tumors requires the production in the neoplastic tissue of a temperature lethal to all cells. A measure of uncertainty still exists about appropriate temperature goals in cryosurgical technique. Certainly cells die in progressively greater numbers as the tissue temperature lowers. Surely also, the cells in a frozen volume of tissue are exposed to diverse thermal profiles, different durations, and the lethality of the freezing of the tissue increases as the temperature falls. Therefore the definition of a targeted temperature goal is important to effectively manage this therapy.

At the beginning of the modern era of cryosurgery, as already mentioned, Cooper's statement, that a tissue temperature of −20°C or colder held for one minute or longer was sufficient to produce necrosis, was soon modified. As cryosurgery was introduced into urological practice in the mid 1960s, Gonder and his associates, who developed the early transurethral freezing technique for prostatic disease, wrote of a freezing time of 8 minutes required to produce a temperature of −40°C in the posterior portion of the prostatic capsule.[37] In this anatomic location, that practice led to untoward complications, such as rectourethal fistula. A few years later, Gonder and his associates recommended that a temperature of −20 to −30°C be produced at the capsule.[38] Other reports of that era suggested even warmer temperatures in order to avoid extra-prostatic freezing and its attendant complications. For example, Dow recommended a prostatic capsular temperature of −10°C and a freezing duration of 7–11 minutes, depending upon the size of the gland, and Green suggested that the capsule temperature be taken only to −6°C in a 4–8 minute period of freezing.[39,40] As the technique of cryosurgery underwent some evolution in the following two decades, few experimental studies of prostate tissue temperatures were reported.[41] However, considerable work on the definition of lethal temperature goals in cryosurgery of other tissues continued.

Because of the paucity of data regarding optimal freezing temperature of the prostate, it is necessary to review data on lethal temperature in other tissues. Using single short freeze–thaw cycles, a number of experiments showed the effect of freezing on the vasculature of skin and mucosa and generally concluded that −20°C was a lethal temperature.[19,42,43] Other investigations with normal tissues or with inoculation of tumor cells in animals have suggested that a tissue temperature of −15 to −20°C was adequate for destruction. For example, experiments with porcine kidneys are cited. Schmidlin and associates, using thermal modeling and correlation with histological findings, set the threshold temperature for complete tissue ablation at −16.1°C.[44] Rupp and associates found the tissue temperature at the border of complete destruction in a single freeze–thaw cycle to be −20°C.[45] Certainly extensive tissue damage occurs in the −20 to −30°C range, but cell destruction in that range is not certain when used for the treatment of tumors, at least not when used in single freeze–thaw cycles.

The tissue temperatures critical for cell death in single freeze–thaw cycles is in the range of −40 to −50°C, as has been shown in experiments with diverse animal tissues.[46–50] These data have been developed under varied experimental conditions: that is, different cells, various freezing times, and several species of animals. Most of the data deal with normal cells rather than cancer cells, which are often more resistant to freezing injury. Some cancer cells are resistant to injury at temperatures of −40°C.[51–54] In experiments with rat prostate tumor tissue, maximal damage was produced at tissue cooling rates greater than 10°C/minute to final temperatures below −40°C. The principal determining factor in tissue destruction was the temperature of −40°C.[33–55] The experiments conducted by Neel and his associates stated that the lethal temperature for animal tumors was −60°C and that repetitive freeze–thaw cycles were required.[56] Cryosurgical research *in vivo* is complex and the injury due to vascular stasis introduces a variable of substantial importance which accounts for the differences in opinion on lethal temperature. Nevertheless, we believe that optimal cell death in clinical applications requires a tissue temperature of −50°C as an appropriate, but approximate, therapeutic goal in the treatment of tumors.

The optimal duration of freezing – that is, how long the tissue should be held in the frozen state – is not known. Some investigators have considered the duration of freezing to be of little importance.[25,53] Indeed, when the tissue temperature is at −40°C and colder, little water remains unfrozen, so the duration is not important. However, when the tissue is held at temperatures warmer than −40°C, especially in the range of −20 to −30°C, recrystallization occurs upon warming, which increases cell destruction. Experiments *in vitro* have shown that frozen cells sustained increased damage when held in the range of −20 to −40°C.[31,53,57] Experiments *in vivo* have demonstrated an increased destructive effect from prolongation of freezing in diverse tissues, including the skin and palate of dogs, the hamster cheek pouch, breast tumors in rats, and the ears of pigs.[20,43,46,58,60] Therefore we and others conclude that holding tissues in the frozen state at a tissue temperature warmer that −40°C will increase destruction.[60]

Slow thawing of the frozen tissue is a prime destructive factor.[26,59–61] The longer the duration of the thawing periods, the greater the damage to the cells because of increased solute effects and maximal growth of ice crystals.[62] The large crystals found during recrystallization produce mechanical disruption of tissues due to an abrasive-like action. Ice crystal growth is especially great at the elevated freezing temperatures, that is, about −20 to −30°C. The thawing of tissue should be done completely and unassisted, which takes full advantage of prolonged hyperosmolality, recrystallization and its attendant effects.

From the beginning of the modern era of cryosurgery, clinical reports have stressed the need for repetitive freezing in cryosurgery for cancer.[2,63,64] Repetition of the freeze–thaw cycle after complete thawing produces more extensive tissue destruction because the cells are subjected to another passage through damaging thermal changes and their attendant deleterious physiochemical effects. In the second freeze–thaw cycle, tissue cooling is faster, the volume of frozen tissue is enlarged, and the border of certain cellular destruction is moved closer to the periphery of the frozen volume of tissue. The disruptive ultrastructural changes in cells are increased with repetition of freezing.[65] The intracellular ice crystals are larger in the second cycle.[66] The disruption of cellular elements and membranes may be responsible for the increase in thermal conductivity evident in tissue in the second cycle.[67]

Research using cells and tissues, and clinical experience have shown the greater destructive effect of repetition of the freeze–thaw cycle.[18,46,54,61,68–76] The enhanced lethal effect is evident at the warmer freezing temperatures near the border of the frozen volume. In this region where the temperature is −30°C or warmer, repetition of freezing enhances destruction. In the central part of the frozen volume, where the tissue temperature is −50°C or colder, a single freeze–thaw cycle is sufficient to destroy the cells.

Practically no attention has been given to the interval between the freeze–thaw cycles, but a delay in the second freezing is almost surely a potential advantage in the direction of increasing destruction. Intracellular ice crystals grow larger with increased time between cooling cycles.[66] The longer the interval between cycles, the greater the failure of the microcirculation. Therefore a delay would increase the efficiency of the second cycle in terms of increased efficacy and more extensive tissue freezing.

The cryogenic lesion is a sharply circumscribed necrosis which closely corresponds to the volume of tissue that was previously frozen. The central portion of the lesion features uniform coagulation necrosis, but the peripheral portion contains dead and viable cells. The closer to the 0°C isotherm at the border of the previously frozen tissue, the greater the number of viable cells. Many cells have the ability to supercool to $-10°C$ or below, so the chance of survival in this temperature range is good.[6] Ultrasound studies have shown that the volume of tissue that became necrotic is somewhat smaller than the volume that was previously frozen.[77] That should be expected because the $-40°C$ isotherm is well within the frozen volume. Infrared thermographic studies during freezing of the skin of rats estimated that the inner 70% of the frozen volume became necrotic.[78] The $-20°C$ isotherm is about 80% of the distance of the ice boundary periphery to the side of the heat sink, the cryoprobe. In the liver, the necrotic tissue is about 80% of the frozen volume when double freeze–thaw cycles are used. Thermal gradients of about 10–15°C/mm are commonly produced in the frozen volume of tissue.

The peripheral portions of the cryogenic lesion, in which the tissue temperature ranged from about 0 to $-40°C$, are of considerable importance to planning therapy. In this region, in which the osmotic stresses are insufficient to cause cell death and intracellular ice crystals are unlikely, a mixture of living and dead cells is found. Recent investigations have identified gene-regulated cell death or apoptosis as a mechanism of cell death in cryosurgery. In an experiment of substantial importance to cryosurgery, Hollister and his associates demonstrated *in vitro* that apoptosis occurs in a wide range of freezing temperatures and continues to as low as $-75°C$.[79] They also showed that the apoptosis could be prevented by an apoptotic inhibitor, which then would permit increased cell survival. Cell death by apoptosis has been noted by other investigators in other tissues.[80–82] Though most of the studies are *in vitro*, experiments have shown that apoptosis occurs *in vivo* also. Wang and associates, working with a glioma in mice, found that apoptosis could be induced by freezing, and that cryochemotherapy enhanced apoptosis.[83] Forest and her associates, in experiments with a non-small-cell cancer xenografted into SCID mice, noted apoptotic cells after freezing. Apoptosis was maximal 8 hours after freezing.[84] The identification of apoptosis as a mechanism of cell death leads to the thought that manipulation of this response may provide a method of increasing the efficacy of cryosurgery.[85] Apoptosis, or programmed cell death, is a genetically regulated process. Apoptotic cell death is activated by a series of molecular and biochemical signaling pathways within a cell in response to an event such as cell stress, nutrient deprivation, growth factor withdrawal, UV radiation, cytotoxic agents, ischemia, and freezing to name a few.[85a] Cells going through apoptosis are characterized by shrinkage, nuclear condensation, loss of mitochondrial potential, activation of cellular proteases (caspases and calpains), non-random DNA fragmentation, cytoplasmic blebbing and the formation of apoptotic bodies. Following the formation of apoptotic bodies *in vivo*, these bodies are phagocytosed by neighboring cells. This series of programmed events is designed to yield cellular destruction in an organized fashion and avoid the activation of an immunologic response to the dying cells.

While there are numerous events which can lead to the activation of apoptosis, there are three primary routes of apoptotic induction including cell surface membrane receptors, the mitochondria, and nuclear activation.[85b] Each of these activation routes results in the recruitment of a host of proteins and enzymes leading to the progression of the apoptotic cascade. While there are a host of activation sites and progression pathways, most pathways converge in the activation of the "caspase cascade" which serves as an amplification process as well as the destructive element of the apoptotic cascade. The "caspase cascade" has been shown to be involved with membrane, mitochondrial, and nuclear-induced apoptosis. Caspase cascade progression typically occurs through the activation of upstream initiator caspases (Caspase 8,9) then the intermediate caspase (i.e. Caspase 4,5,6) followed by activation of the execution caspases (Caspase 3 and 7), which result in cleavage of target proteins such as PARP (poly(ADP-ribose)polymerase) and IAP (inhibitor of apoptosis) which in turn result in DNA cleavage and cell death.

While much is known about apoptosis, there is little known about the mechanisms of action and progression as a result of freezing injury. Recently a study by Clarke et al[31] implicated the role of mitochondria in the activation of freeze-induced apoptosis. Additional studies in the freeze injury model of cryopreservation have shown that there is an activation of the membrane-associated apoptotic mechanism as well as the mitochondrial-dependent events.[86] Investigation into the mechanisms of activation continue with new reports emerging steadily. In fact, very recent work by Clarke et al (unpublished) has revealed the role of cell cycle disruption and stress response pathway activation following freezing injury in apoptotic induction. As these studies continue, our knowledge base will continue to expand and provide further understanding into the mode, mechanisms, and timing of cell death following freezing injury.

IMPLICATIONS FOR CLINICAL TECHNIQUE

The basic features of cryosurgical technique for the treatment of tumors have long been recognized as fast cooling to a lethal temperature, slow thawing, and repetition of the freeze–thaw cycle. In general, the cryosurgical probe is always used as cold as possible because a large thermal gradient is needed to freeze a volume of tissue as quickly as can be achieved and to produce a lethal temperature at some distance from the heat sink provided by the probe. When the probe is used as cold as possible, as is usually the case, the rate of cooling and freezing are fixed and depend upon the heat transfer characteristics of the probe. The freezing capability of a probe depends upon its temperature, the surface area for heat transfer, and the thermal conductivity of the probe/cryogen. Tissue conductivity is not of practical importance in cryosurgery because most tissues have a high water content and the cooling efficiency of the apparatus is sufficient for almost all tissues.[87]

In clinical practice, though the basic features of cryosurgical technique for tumors have been well accepted, deviations from optimal technique are common. These deviations are prompted in part by the time required to complete the surgery, and also by anatomical constraints in some areas, such as the prostate gland. The clinician must be concerned with the risk/benefits of changing these long-accepted basic tenets. A common deviation is in the choice of temperature goals. A tissue temperature of $-20°C$ has been thought adequate by some investigators.[44,45] Extensive tissue damage occurs at this temperature, but certainty of cell destruction is not likely. A tissue temperature goal of $-40°C$ in the normal tissue about 1 cm beyond the apparent limits of the cancer will provide a margin of safety comparable to surgical excision in most types of neoplasms. This recommendation is not practical in some anatomic locations, such as the proximity of the rectum to the prostate capsule. Therefore in the cryosurgical treatment of prostatic cancer, in order to avoid freezing the rectum, a temperature end point of -20 to $-30°C$ is used at the prostatic capsule so that the rectum is not injured.[88] The use of repetitive freezing techniques might suffice for $-20°C$, especially if held at that temperature for several minutes. Nevertheless, the more efficacious technique, given measures to protect the rectum and urethral sphincters, would be to use a double freeze–thaw cycle and a tissue temperature of $-40°C$.[89,90] The same technique should be used for kidney tumors.[91] One possible solution to this problem would be to rely on the differential sensitivity of human cells to low temperatures along with the use of adjunctive protective agents in the rectum.

Another questionable practice is the use of single freeze–thaw cycles. Certainly in experiments with normal tissues, such as the kidney, single freeze–thaw cycles do substantial damage to the tissue. However, cancer cells often survive single freeze–thaw cycles. Therefore the use of a single freeze–thaw cycle is generally not advisable for cancer therapy. In clinical practice, repeated freeze–thaw cycles are used in several ways. The optimal technique is to repeat the cycle after a complete thawing of the tissue. However, in the technique commonly used in the prostate and liver, only a partial thaw is permitted, so that the probes are not dislodged. The effect is to repeat freezing of only the peripheral zones, which may be sufficient for therapy since that is the region where the chance of cell survival is greater.

A third variation in practice is the thaw time. Woolley and associates, following experiments *in vivo*, recommended a double freeze–thaw cycle, but advocated an active thaw in order to reduce operative time.[75] Warming a cold probe is commonly needed to change its position, but the entire lesion should not be thawed actively. Nevertheless the thawing period has bidirectional characteristics, whether active or passive. Once the probe is inactivated, the iceball becomes the heat sink and warms from the probe outward and the iceball radius inward. In the matter of a passive thaw, the heat flux from the probe would be minimal compared with that radiating from the radius. It might, over a few minutes, be adequate to melt the probe–iceball interface supporting probe extraction. The thawing period is also affected by use of the techniques to protect important tissue, such as the use of warming solutions to protect the urethra during prostatic freezing. The application of a rapid thaw with a heated probe may create a "rescue" condition for partially damaged cells.

The results of cryosurgical treatment have improved as greater experience with the techniques has been gained and improved imaging techniques have evolved, perhaps also as concomitant use of thermocouples has become more common. Nevertheless, the results are susceptible to further improvement. The incidence of persistent (recurring) disease after cryotherapy for prostatic cancer varies with case selection and with different physicians, but generally is about 10–30%, as manifested by prostate specific antigen levels and prostatic biopsies several years after cryosurgery.[92–95] In the treatment of liver tumors the incidence of persistent cancer in the cryo-treated site ranges from 10 to 40%.[96,97] Experience with the cryosurgical treatment of kidney tumors is relatively recent with rather small numbers of patients having been treated. It seems likely that a persistent rate of 5–10% will be found with longer follow-up.[91,98–100] The incidence of persistent tumors in cryo-treated sites shows the need for improvement in the technique or in selection of patients. Rukstalis and his associates have defined some directions for modification of prostatic cryoablation which should improve efficacy.[101] Some failures are due to less-than-optimal freezing technique and some may be due to errors in judgment about the extent of disease, which may be due to interpretation of the images. Putting those reasons aside, the failures show the need for adjunctive therapy.

To increase the chance of cure, adjunctive therapy is needed to increase the rate and the completeness of cell death in the periphery of the cryogenic lesion. Adjunctive therapy may include several agents, including cancer chemotherapeutic drugs, irradiation, or other chemical agents. The use of androgen ablation therapy before cryosurgery is an adjunctive therapeutic modality also, but we focus on the agents to increase the lethal effect of freezing. Cancer chemotherapeutic drugs are the most commonly used adjunctive agents, and are considered to be beneficial. The timing of the administration of the drug is not well known. Commonly the drug has been given before or after cryosurgery, but usage has not been integrated with the freezing in an orderly manner. A measure of caution is needed regarding dosage, especially when used as an adjunct to cryosurgery of hepatic tumors. When the usual customary doses are used, the combined effect of chemotherapy and cryosurgery may lead to coagulopathy when large volumes of tissue are frozen. This is not likely to happen in cryosurgery of the kidney or prostate gland, in part because the volume of tissue frozen is relatively small in comparison to that often required for hepatic neoplasms. One strategy for the use of chemotherapy might be to avoid the timing issue and use a metronomic schedule. Continuous low-dose chemotherapy is thought to inhibit tumor angiogenesis, which is a critical need in the growth of tumors. Metronomic therapy has been advantageous in diverse tumors.[102,103] This style of drug therapy may be especially effective in prostatic cancer because in the majority of cases, the cells proliferate slowly, so resistance to the many drugs that target dividing cells is common.

Anti-cancer drugs are likely to be helpful in promoting cell death in the periphery of the previously frozen tissues, probably by apoptosis, as has been suggested by the experiments *in vitro* of Clarke and his associates.[31] They showed that in human prostate cancer cells (PCA) a combination of freezing and 5-fluorouracil produced a greater reduction in cell survival than either freezing or the drug alone. Their later experiments demonstrated an increase in pro-apoptotic Bax protein levels following a cryochemotherapy combination, including 5-fluorouracil and capsulation.[104] The potential for benefit was demonstrated also by the experiments of Wang and his associates, working with mouse models with glioma cells, which showed enhancement of apoptosis by cryochemotherapy.[83]

Cancer chemotherapeutic drugs can be concentrated in the tumor area by an appropriately timed delivery.[105] Intravenous administration of the drug during cryosurgery will result in a high long-lasting concentration of the drug in the tumor area as microcirculatory failure develops after thawing.[106,107] Since freezing alters membrane permeability, entry of the drug into the cell may be facilitated, as has been shown to be true for bleomycin in the experiments of Mir and Rubinsky.[108] Drugs also can be injected directly into the tumor during the period of thawing without gaining significant entry into the general circulation. Local chemotherapy also may be given directly into the tumor by placing the anticancer agent on a carrier, which then is placed into the track left after removal of the cryoprobe. This would allow slow absorption of the agent, yet with little access to the general blood circulation. LePivert and his associates have demonstrated some benefit to this approach in experimental work.[109]

Radiotherapy is commonly used in the course of many tumors treated also by cryosurgery. However, as is true of chemotherapy, the appropriate time of delivery has never been established. Experiments *in vitro* have demonstrated that the sensitivity of cooled cells to irradiation is increased.[110,111] Perhaps adjunctive radiotherapy at an appropriate time would be beneficial. One would expect radiotherapy to promote apoptosis in the peripheral area of the cryolesion and thus, increase the chance of cure.

Other agents, such as antifreeze proteins and apoptosis-promoting drugs, may prove useful in adjunctive therapy. Antifreeze proteins are glycoproteins that can induce ice crystal formations and enhance the destructive effects of freezing.[112,113] Experiments *in vivo* have demonstrated enhanced cell destruction by injection of antifreeze proteins into tumors.[114] The apoptosis-promoting drugs have increased damage from freezing injury in cell suspensions.[115] Tumor necrosis factor (TNF) has a toxic effect on tumor vasculature.[116] Experiments *in vivo*, using a human prostate subline, showed that the local use of TNF-alpha enhanced the inflammatory response to freezing and increased the degree of injury, probably via the vascular failure mechanism.[117] None of these agents has had a clinical trial. Some newer therapies, such as angiogenesis inhibitors, currently being evaluated for the treatment of advanced prostatic cancer, may be useful as adjuncts to cryosurgical treatment.[118]

As adjunctive therapeutic agents, immunologic-enhancing drugs must also be considered. The concept of cryoimmunology has a long history in relation to prostatic disease. Shulman and his associates in 1967 suggested that freezing prostatic cancer *in situ* would elicit a beneficial response.[119] Prostatic cryosurgery repeated at intervals of a few weeks was thought to elicit a booster response.[38] Since than many investigations have been directed at the nature of the immunologic response. Several investigations have shown benefit from an immunologic response in experimental tumors.[120–122] Others have found no evidence of benefit in a prostate cancer cell line.[123] Immunologic-enhancing drugs have been used experimentally and clinically, and have been considered helpful.[124–127] Nevertheless, evidence of clear benefit in human tumors is lacking. One should recognize that the cryoimmunologic response has another facet. In one animal study, freezing tumors *in situ* has provoked enhanced metastases.[128] In animals and in humans, the cytokine release after freezing has caused deleterious inflammatory responses in important organs, especially after freezing large volumes of tissue.[129–132] Nevertheless interest in cryoimmunology is quite high, so perhaps some applications may be found in the future.

SUMMARY

Cryosurgery is a sophisticated therapy that subjects the cancer to a cascade of destructive stresses, such as ice crystal formation, post-thaw necrosis due to partial ice-related damage, apoptosis due to multiple oxidative stress, and then coagulative necrosis due to vascular stasis. Physical processes of destruction are effective immediately, physiological-based destruction related to stress at the cellular level occurs over hours to days, and sequelae related to vascular damage, cytokine release, provide damaging effects over many days. To fully exploit these facets of injury and to achieve therapeutic efficacy demands careful attention to the freeze–thaw cycles.

The basic principles of cryosurgery for tumors are fast freezing the tissue to an appropriate level, slow thawing, and repetition of the freeze–thaw cycle. Ideally a temperature of $-40°C$ in the normal tissue around a tumor should be the goal. The incidence of persistent disease in cryo-treated sites in diverse organs suggests that current application of these principles may not be optimal. In part this is due to anatomical constraints, especially for example the proximity of the prostate gland to the rectum. The limitations of cryosurgery emphasize the importance of the use of adjunctive therapy or molecular-based therapy in some form in order to influence the fate of the cells in the peripheral zone of the cryolesion. A better understanding of the molecular mechanisms involved in cryogenic injury and adjunct therapy, targeting specific molecular pathways, is expected to lead to enhanced efficacy of cryosurgical technique.

REFERENCES

1. Cooper IS. Cryobiology as viewed by the surgeon. Cryobiology 1964; 1: 44–51.
2. Cooper IS. Cryogenic surgery for cancer. Fed Proc 1965; 24: S237–40.
3. Kreyberg L. Tissue damage due to cold. Lancet 1946; 1: 338–40.
4. Mazur P. Freezing of living cells: mechanisms and implications. Am J Physiol 1984; 143: C125–42.
5. Muldrew K, McGann LE. The osmotic rupture hypothesis of intracellular freezing injury. Biophys J 1994; 66: 532–41.
6. Mazur P. Physical-chemical factors underlying cell injury in cryosurgical freezing. In: Rand R, Rinfret A, VonLeden H, eds. Cryosurgery. Springfield, II: Charles C Thomas, 1967: 32–51.
7. Toscano WM, Cravalho EG, Silvares OM, Huggins CE. The thermodynamics of intracellular ice nucleation in the freezing of erythrocytes. J Heat Transfer 1975; 97: 326–32.
8. Rubinsky B, Lee CY, Bastacky J, Onik G. The process of freezing and the mechanism of damage during hepatic cryosurgery. Cryobiology 1990; 27: 85–97.
9. Bischof JC, Cristov K, Rubinsky B. A morphological study of the cooling rate response of normal and neoplastic liver tissue. Cryobiology 1993; 30: 482–92.
10. Hong J, Rubinsky B. Patterns of ice formation in normal and malignant breast tissue. Cryobiology 1994; 31: 109–20.
11. Berger WK, Uhrik B. Freeze-induced shrinkage of individual cells and cell-to-cell propagation of intracellular ice in cell chains from salivary glands. Experientia 1996; 52: 843–50.
12. Mundth ED. Studies on the pathogenesis of cold injury: microcirculatory changes in tissue injured by freezing. Proc Symp Artic Biol Med 1964; 4: 51–72.
13. Quintanella R, Krusen F, Essex H. Studies on frostbite with special reference to treatment and the effect on minute blood vessels. Am J Physiol 1947; 149: 149–61.
14. Zacarian S, Stone D, Clater M. Effects of cryogenic temperatures on microcirculation in the golden hamster cheek pouch. Cryobiology 1970; 7: 27–39.
15. Bellman S, Ray JA. Vascular reactions after experimental cold injury. Angiology 1956; 7: 339–67.
16. Bowers WD, Hubbard RW, Daum RC, Ashbaugh P, Nilson E et al. Ultrastructural studies of muscle cells and vascular endothelium immediately after freeze–thaw injury. Cryobiology 1973; 10: 9–21.
17. Giampapa V, Oh C, Aufses A. The vascular effect of cold injury. Cryobiology 1981; 18: 49–54.
18. Gill W, DaCosta J, Fraser J. The control and predictability of a cryolesion. Cryobiology 1970; 6: 347–53.
19. LaFebvre JH, Folke LE. Effects of subzero temperatures on the microcirculation in the oral mucous membrane. Microvasc Res 1975; 10: 360–72.
20. Lenz M. Cryosurgery of the cheek pouch of the golden Syrian hamster. Int Surg 1972; 57: 223–8.
21. Ninomiya T, Yosimura H, Mori M. Identification of vascular system in experimental carcinoma for cryosurgery – histochemical observations of lectin UEA-1 and alkaline phosphatase activity in vascular endothelium. Cryobiology 1985; 33: 331–5.
22. Rabb JM, Renaud ML, Brandt A, Witt CW. Effect of freezing and thawing on the microcirculation and capillary endothelium of hamster cheek pouch. Cryobiology 1974; 11: 508–18.
23. Rothenberg H. Cutaneous circulation in rabbit and humans before, during, and after cryosurgical procedures, measured by Xenon-133 clearance. Cryobiology 1970; 6: 507–11.
24. Whittaker D. Vascular response in oral mucosa following cryosurgery. J Periodont Res 1977; 12: 55–63.
25. Whittaker D. Electron microscopy of the ice crystals formed during cryosurgery: relationship to duration of freeze. Cryobiology 1978; 15: 603–7.

26. Whittaker DK. Mechanisms of tissue destruction following cryosurgery. Ann R Coll Surg England 1984; 66: 313–18.
27. Bourne MH, Piepkern MW, Clayton F, Leonard LG. Analysis of microvascular changes in frostbite injury. J Surg Res 1986; 40: 26–35.
28. Gage AA, Ishikawa H, Winter PM. Experimental frostbite and hyperbaric oxygenation. Surgery 1969; 66: 1044–50.
29. Hoffman NE, Bischof JC. Cryosurgery of normal and tumor tissue in the dorsal skin flap chamber: part II – injury response. Tissue ASME 1981; 123: 310–16.
30. LePivert P. Basic considerations of the cryolesion. In: Ablin R, ed. Cryosurgery. New York: Dekker, 1980: 15–68.
31. Clarke DM, Baust JM, Van Buskirk RG, Baust JG. Chemo-cryo combination therapy: an adjunctive model for the treatment of prostate cancer. Cryobiology 2001; 42: 274–85.
32. Baust JG, Gage AA, Ma H, Zhang CM. Minimally invasive cryosurgery – technological advances. Cryobiology 1997; 34: 373–84.
33. Bischof JC, Smith D, Pazhayannur PV et al. Cryosurgery of Dunning AT-1 rat prostate tumor: thermal, biophysical, and viability response at the cellular and tissue level. Cryobiology 1997; 34: 42–69.
34. Hong J, Rubinsky B. Patterns of ice formation in normal and malignant breast tissue. Cryobiology 1994; 31: 109–20.
35. Whittaker DK. Ice crystals formed in tissue during cryosurgery. I. Light microscopy. Cryobiology 1974; 11: 192–201.
36. Farrant J, Walter CA. The cryobiological basis for cryosurgery. J Derm Surg Oncol 1977; 3: 403–7.
37. Gonder M, Soanes W, Shulman S. Cryosurgical treatment of the prostate. Invest Urol 1966; 3: 372–8.
38. Soanes W, Gonder M. Cryosurgery in benign and malignant disease of the prostate. Int Surg 1969; 51: 104–16.
39. Dow J. Effects of surgical capsular temperature on cryosurgery of the prostate. J Urol 1968; 100: 66–71.
40. Green N. Cryosurgery of the prostate gland. Ann Royal Coll Surg Engl 1977; 59: 288–97.
41. Gage AA, Huben R. Cryosurgical ablation of the prostate. Urol Oncol 2000; 5: 11–19.
42. Lenz H, Goertz G, Preussler H. The minimal freezing temperatures for a necrosis of the epidermis and the influence of cryoprotective agents. Arch Oto-Rhino-Laryngol 1975; 209: 217–21.
43. Zacarian S, Stone D, Clater M. Effects of cryogenic temperatures on microcirculation in the golden hamster cheek pouch. Cryobiology 1970; 7: 27–39.
44. Schmidlin FR, Rupp CC, Hoffmann NE et al. Measurement and prediction of thermal behavior and acute assessment of injury in a pig model of renal cryosurgery. J Endourol 2001; 15: 193–7.
45. Rupp CC, Hoffmann NE, Schmidlin FR et al. Cryosurgical changes in the porcine kidney: histologic analysis with thermal history correlation. Cryobiology 2002; 45: 167–82.
46. Gage AA. Experimental cryogenic injury of the palate: observations pertinent to the cryosurgical destruction of tumors. Cryobiology 1978; 15: 415–25.
47. Gage AA. What temperature is lethal for cells? J Dermatol Surg 1979; 5: 459–61.
48. Staren ED, Sobel MS, Gianakakis LM et al. Cryosurgery of breast cancer. Arch Surg 1997; 132: 28–33.
49. Yamada S, Tsubouchi S. Rapid cell death and cell population recovery in mouse skin epidermis after freezing. Cryobiology 1976; 13: 317–27.
50. El-Shakha SA, Shimi SA, Cuschieri A. Effective hepatic cryoablation: does it enhance tumor dissemination? World J Surg 1999; 23: 306–10.
51. Heard BE. Nuclear crystals in slowly frozen tissues at very low temperatures: comparison of normal and ascites tumour cells. Br J Surg 1955; 42: 659–63.
52. Zacarian SA. The observation of freeze–thaw cycles upon cancer cell suspensions. J Dermat Surg Oncol 1977; 3: 173–4.

53. Jacob G, Kurzer MN, Fuller BJ. An assessment of tumor cell viability after *in vitro* freezing. Cryobiology 1985; 22: 417–26.
54. Tatsutani K, Rubinsky B, Onik G, Dahiya R. The effect of thermal variables on frozen human prostatic adenocarcinoma cells. Urology 1996; 48: 441–7.
55. Roberts KP, Smith DJ, Ozturi H et al. Biochemical alterations and tissue viability in AT-1 prostate tumor tissue after *in vitro* cryodestruction. Cryo-Lett 1997; 10: 241–50.
56. Neel HB 3rd, Ketchum AS, Hammond WG. Requisites for successful cryogenic surgery of cancer. Arch Surg 1971; 102: 45–8.
57. Rubinsky B. The freezing process and mechanism of tissue damage. In: Onik GM, Rubinsky B, Watson G, Ablin RJ. eds. Percutaneous Prostate Cryoablation St. Louis: Quality Medical Publishing, 1995: 49–68.
58. Burge SM, Shepherd JP, Dawber RPR. Effect of freezing the helix and edge of the human and pig ear. J Dermatol Surg Oncol 1984; 10: 816–19.
59. Gage AA, Guest K, Montes M, Caruana JA et al. Effect of varying freezing and thawing rates in experimental cryosurgery. Cryobiology 1985; 22: 175–82.
60. Hoffmann NE, Bischof JC. The cryobiology of cryosurgical injury. Urology 2002; 60: 40–9.
61. Neel HB, DeSanto LW. Cryosurgical control of cancer. Effects of freeze rates, tumor temperatures, and ischemia. Ann Otol 1973; 82: 716–23.
62. Mazur P. The role of intracellular freezing in the death of cells cooled at supraoptimal rates. Cryobiology 1977; 14: 251–72.
63. Cahan W. Cryosurgery of malignant and benign tumors. Fed Proc 1965; 24: S241–8.
64. Gage AA, Koepf S, Wehrle D, Emmings F. Cryotherapy for cancer of the lip and oral cavity. Cancer 1965; 18: 1646–51.
65. Gill W, Fraser J, Carter D. Repeated freeze–thaw cycles in cryosurgery. Nature 1968; 239: 410–13.
66. Whittaker DK. Repeat freeze cycles in cryosurgery of oral tissues. Br Dent J 1975; 139: 459–65.
67. Poppendiek HP, Randall FR, Breeden JA, Chambers JE, Murphy JR et al. Thermal conductivity measurements and predictions for biological fluids and tissues. Cryobiology 1967; 4: 318–27.
68. Gage AA, Caruana JA, Montes M. Critical temperature for skin necrosis in experimental cryosurgery. Cryobiology 1982; 19: 273–82.
69. Gage AA, Augustynowicz S, Montes M et al. Tissue impedance and temperature measurements in relation to necrosis in experimental cryosurgery. Cryobiology 1985; 22: 282–8.
70. Myers RS, Hammond WG, Ketcham AS. Cryosurgery of experimental tumors. J Cryosurg 1969; 2: 225–8.
71. Neel HB, Ketcham AS, Hammond WG. Cryonecrosis of normal and tumor-bearing rat liver potentiated by inflow occlusion. Cancer 1971; 28: 1211–18.
72. Rand RW, Rand RP, Eggerding F, DenBesten L, King W. Cryolumpectomy for carcinoma of the breast. Surg Gynecol Obstet 1987; 165: 392–6.
73. Ravikumar TS, Steele G, Kane R, King V. Experimental and clinical observations on hepatic cryosurgery for colorectal metastases. Cancer Res 1991; 31: 6323–7.
74. Dilley AV, Dy DY, Warlters A et al. Laboratory and animal model evaluations of the Cryotech LCS 2000 in hepatic cryosurgery. Cryobiology 1993; 30: 74–85.
75. Woolley M, Schulsinger DA, Durand DB, Zeltser IS, Waltzer WC. Effect of freezing parameters (freeze cycle and thaw process) on tissue destruction following renal cryoablation. J Endourol 2002; 16: 519–22.
76. Mala T, Edwin B, Tillung T et al. Percutaneous cryoablation of colorectal liver metastases: potentiated by two consecutive freeze–thaw cycles. Cryobiology 2003; 46: 99–102.
77. Saliken JC, Cohen J, Miller R, Robert M. Laboratory evaluation of ice formation around a 3-mm Accuprobe. Cryobiology 1995; 32: 285–95.
78. Pogrel MA, Yen CK, Taylor R. A study of infrared thermographic assessment of liquid nitrogen cryotherapy. Oral Surg Oral Med Oral Pathol Oral Radiol Endod 1996; 81: 396–401.

79. Hollister WR, Mathew AJ, Baust JG, Van Buskirk RG. Effects of freezing on cell viability and mechanisms of cell death in a human prostate cancer cell line. Mol Urol 1998; 2: 13–18.
80. Hanai A, Yang WI, Ravikumar TS. Induction of apoptosis in human colon carcinoma cells HT29 by sublethal cryo-injury: mediation by cytochrome-c release. Int J Cancer 2001; 93: 526–33.
81. Yang WI, Addona T, Nair DG, Lixin Q, Ravikumar TS. Apoptosis induced by cryo-injury in human colorectal cancer cells is associated with mitochondrial dysfunction. Int J Cancer 2003; 103: 360–9.
82. Steinbach JP, Weissenberger J, Aguzzi A. Distinct phases of cryogenic tissue damage in the cerebral cortex of wild-type and c-fos deficient mice. Neuropathol Appl Neurobiol 1999; 25: 468–80.
83. Wang H, Tu HJ, Qin J et al. Effects of cryotherapy and 5-fluorouacil on apoptosis of G422 glioma cells. AiZheng 2004; 23: 412–15. (in Chinese)
84. Forest V. Peoc'h M, Camos L, Guyotat D, Vergnon JM. Effects of cryotherapy or chemotherapy on apoptosis in a non-small-cell cancer xenografted into SCID mice. Cryobiology 2005; 50: 29–37.
85. Baust JG, Gage AA, Clarke D, Baust JM, Van Buskirk RG. Cryosurgery – a putative approach to molecular-based optimization. Cryobiology 2004; 48: 190–204.
85a. Baust JM. Molecular mechanisms of cellular demise associated with cryopreservation failure. Cell Preserv Technol 2002; 1: 17–32.
85b. Edinger AL, Thompson CB. Death by design: apoptosis necrosis and autophagy. Curr Opin in Cell Biol 2004; 16: 663–9.
86. Baust JM, Van Buskirk R, Baust JG. Generation activation of the apoptotic cascade following cryogenic storage. Cell Preserv Technol 2002; 1: 63–80.
87. Ponder E. The coefficient of thermal conductivity of blood and various tissues. J Gen Physiol 1962; 45: 545–51.
88. Onik O. Cryosurgery. Crit Rev Oncol Hematol 1996; 23: 1–24.
89. Wong WS, Chinn DO, Chinn M et al. Cryosurgery as a treatment for prostate carcinoma: results and complications. Cancer 1997; 79: 963–74.
90. Larson TR, Robertson DW, Corica A, Bostwick DG. *In vivo* interstitial temperature mapping of the human prostate during cryosurgery with correlation to histopathologic outcomes. Urology 2000; 55: 547–52.
91. Rukstalis DB, Khorsandi M, Garcia FU, Hoenig DM, Cohen JK. Clinical experience with open renal cryoablation. Urology 2001; 57: 34–9.
92. Donnelly BJ, Saliken JC, Ernst DS et al. Prospective trial of cryosurgical ablation of the prostate: five-year results. Urology 2002; 60: 645–9.
93. Han KR, Cohen JK, Miller RJ et al. Treatment of organ confined prostate cancer with third generation cryosurgery: preliminary multicenter experience. J Urol 2003; 170: 1126–30.
94. Long JP, Bahn D, Lee F, Shinohara K et al. Five-year retrospective, multi-institutional pooled analysis of cancer-related outcomes after cryosurgical ablation of the prostate. Urology 2001; 57: 518–23.
95. Katz AE, Rewcastle JC. The current and potential role of cryoablation as a primary therapy for localized prostate cancer. Curr Oncol Rep 2003; 5: 231–8.
96. Seifert JK, Junginger T, Morris DL. Collective review of world literature on hepatic cryosurgery. J R Coll Surg Ed 1998; 43: 141–54.
97. Seifert JK, Junginger T. Cryotherapy for liver tumors: current status, perspectives, clinical results, and review of literature. Technol Cancer Res Treat 2004; 3: 151–63.
98. Lee DI, McGinnis DE, Feld R, Strup SE. Retroperitoneal laparoscopic cryoablation of small renal tumors: intermediate results. Urology 2003; 61: 83–8.
99. Nadler RB, Kim SC, Rubenstein JN et al. Laparoscopic renal cryosurgery: the Northwestern experience. J Urol 2003; 170: 1121–5.
100. Spaliviero M, Moinzadeh A, Gill IS. Laparoscopic cryotherapy for renal tumors. Technol Cancer Res Treat 2004; 3: 177–80.

101. Rukstalis DB, Goldknopf JL, Crowley EM, Garcia FU. Prostate cryoablation A scientific rationale for future modifications. Urology 2002; 60: 19–25.
102. Glode LM, Barqawi A, Crighton F, Crawford ED, Kerbel R. Metronomic therapy with cyclophosphamide and dexamethasone for prostate carcinoma. Cancer 2003; 98: 1643–8.
103. Drevs J, Fakler J, Eisele S et al. Antiangiogenic potency of various chemotherapeutic drugs for metronomic chemotherapy. Anticancer Res 2004; 24: 1759–63.
104. Clarke DM, Baust JM, Van Buskirk RG, Baust JG. Addition of anticancer agents enhances freezing-induced prostate cancer cell death: implication of mitochondrial involvement. Cryobiology 2004; 49: 45–61.
105. Benson JW. Regional chemotherapy and cryotherapy for cancer. Oncology 1972; 26: 134–51.
106. Ikekewa S, Ishihara K, Tanaka S, Ikeda S. Basic studies of cryochemotherapy in a murine tumor system. Cryobiology 1985; 22: 477–83.
107. Homasson JP, Pecking A, Robert S, Angebault M, Bennoit JP. Tumor fixation of bleomycin labeled with 57 cobalt before and after cryotherapy of bronchial carcinoma. Cryobiology 1992; 29: 543–8.
108. Mir LM, Rubinsky B. Treatment of cancer with cryochemotherapy. Br J Cancer 2002; 86: 1658–60.
109. LePivert P, Haddad RS, Aller A et al. Ultrasound guided combined cryoablation and microencapsulated 5-fluorouracil inhibits growth of human prostate tumors in xenogenic mouse model assessed by luminescence imaging. Technol Cancer Res Treat 2004; 3: 135–42.
110. Burton SA, Paljug WR, Kalmicki S, Werts ED. Hypothermic enhanced human tumor cell radiosensitivity. Cryobiology 1997; 35: 70–8.
111. Znati CA, Werts E, Kociban D, Kalnicki S. Variables influencing response of human prostate carcinoma cells to combined radiation and cryotherapy *in vitro*. Cryobiology 1998; 37: 450–1.
112. Koushafer H, Rubinsky B. Effects of antifreeze proteins on frozen primary prostatic adenocarcinoma cells. Urology 1997; 49: 421–5.
113. Pham I, Dahiya R, Rubinsky B. An *in vivo* study of antifreeze protein adjuvant cryosurgery. Cryobiology 1999; 38: 169–75.
114. Muldrew K, Rewcastle J, Donnelly BJ et al. Flounder antifreeze peptides increase the efficacy of cryosurgery. Cryobiology 2001; 42: 182–9.
115. Clarke DM, Hollister WR, Baust JG, Van Buskirk RG. Cryosurgical modeling: sequence of freezing and cytotoxic agent application affects cell death. Mol Urol 1999; 3: 25–31.
116. Watanabe M, Niitsu Y, Umeno H et al. Toxic effect of tumor necrosis factor on tumor vasculature in mice. Cancer Res 1988; 48: 2179–83.
117. Choe BH, He X, Bischof JC. Pretreatment inflammation induced by TNF-alpha augments cryosurgical injury on human prostate cancer. Cryobiology 2004; 49: 10–27.
118. Hegeman RB, Liu G, Wilding G, McNeel DG. Newer therapies in advanced prostate cancer. Clin Prostate Cancer 2004; 3: 150–6.
119. Shulman S, Yantorno C, Bronson P. Cryoimmunology: a method of immunization to autologous tissue. Proc Soc Exp Biol Med 1967; 124: 658–66.
120. Blackwood CE, Cooper IS. Response of experimental tumor systems to cryosurgery. Cryobiology 1972; 9: 508–15.
121. Joosten JJ, van Muijen GN, Wobbes T et al. *In vivo* destruction of tumor tissue by cryoablation can induce inhibition of secondary tumor growth: an experimental study. Cryobiology 2001; 42: 49–58.
122. Joosten JJ, van Muijen GN, Wobbes T, Ruers TJ. Cryosurgery of tumor tissue causes endotoxin tolerance through an inflammatory response. Anticancer Res 2003; 23: 427–32.
123. Hoffmann NE, Coad JF, Huot CS, Swanlund DJ, Bischof JC. Investigation of the mechanism and the effect of cryoimmunology in the Copenhagen rat. Cryobiology 2001; 42: 59–68.
124. Shibata T, Suzuki K, Yamashita T et al. Immunological analysis of enhanced spontaneous metastasis in WKA rats following cryosurgery. Anticancer Res 1998; 18: 2483–6.

125. Slovin SF, Kelly WK, Scher HI. Immunological approaches for the treatment of prostate cancer. Semin Urol Oncol 1998; 16: 53–9.
126. Bremers AJ, Kuppen PJ, Parmiani X. Tumor immunotherapy: the adjuvant treatment of the 21st century? Eur J Surg Oncol 2000; 26: 418–24.
127. Urano M, Tanaka C, Sugiyama Y, Miya K, Saji S. Antitumor effects of residual tumor after cryoablation: the combined effect of residual tumor and a protein-bound polysaccharide on multiple liver metastases in a murine model. Cryobiology 2003; 46: 238–45.
128. Yamashita T, Hayakawa K, Hosokawa M et al. Enhanced tumor metastases in rats following cryosurgery of primary tumor. Gann 1982; 73: 222–8.
129. Seifert JK, France MP, Zhao J et al. Large volume hepatic freezing: association with significant release of the cytokine interleukin-5 and tumor necrosis factor in a rat model. World J Surg 2002; 26: 1333–41.
130. Fushimi N, Jinno O, Washida H, Ueda K, Otaguro K. Humoral immunity following double-freezing of the prostate in patients with prostate cancer. Cryobiology 1982; 19: 242–6.
131. Chapman WC, Debelak JP, Blackwell TS et al. Cyroablation-induced acute lung injury: pulmonary hemodynamic and permeability effects in a sheep model. Arch Surg 2000; 135: 667–72.
132. Wudel IJ Jr, Allos TM, Washington MK, Sheller JR, Chapman WC. Multi-organ inflammation after hepatic cryoablation in BALB/c mice. J Surg Res 2003; 112: 131–7.

2

The evolution of cryotherapy for localized prostate cancer

Michael J. Manyak

Introduction • Early prostate cryotherapy • Development of modern cryotherapy
• Future of cryotherapy

INTRODUCTION

The recognition that very cold temperature will destroy soft tissue is an old concept that had very limited applications in medicine until relatively recent imaging technology allowed more precise access to lesions other than superficial epithelial tumors. In conjunction with enhanced imaging, the practical application of cryoablation required technological development of other key components such as the freezing agent, the delivery mechanism, and the technique of safe and efficient treatment. Cryoablation was not considered as a potential treatment option for prostate disease until there was synergy with all of these components.

A comprehensive review of cryotherapeutic history is beyond the scope of this chapter and the interested reader is referred to excellent reviews of this development published elsewhere.[1,2] However, a brief chronological synopsis of this modality illustrates the various stages of development beginning with the early reports of James Arnott in the mid 1800s. Arnott was one of the first to publicize the use of saline solutions of crushed ice (reaching $-24°C$) as a topical anesthetic. Over the next century, cryogenic agents and various cryosurgical techniques were used sporadically for diverse medical applications including eradication of tumors in several organs.

The next practical expansion of clinical application occurred just before 1900 when liquefied gases were shown to provide significantly colder temperatures suitable for more extensive tissue effects. Early approaches were limited to direct superficial applications of either the cryogenic agent (usually liquid nitrogen) or an inert cooled metal disc to the surface of a lesion. Though limited in scope, some of these original applications, such as destruction of dermatological lesions, persist in clinical use today.[3]

Cryotherapy began to enter the modern world in 1961 with the introduction of an advanced liquid nitrogen cryogenic probe by Cooper and Lee.[4] For the first time, effective, controlled, and deep tissue freezing was accomplished with the small-caliber, vacuum-insulated, multi-lumen cryogenic probe that closely resembled modern liquid cryoprobes.

EARLY PROSTATE CRYOTHERAPY

One of the first reports of prostate cryotherapy for bladder neck obstruction from benign and malignant disease occurred in 1966.[5] Gonder and Soanes used a single, blunt-end, transurethral cryoprobe and monitored the freezing progress by digital palpation from the rectum, augmented usually by a thermosensor needle in Denonvilliers' space. Refinement of the procedure to improve efficacy combined transurethral freezing with an open perineal approach to expose the prostatic apex and separate and protect the rectum.[6] Although sufficient cancer control prompted further development, this approach was limited due to complications of significant urinary dysfunction and urethral sloughing. Cryotherapy for obstruction from benign prostatic hyperplasia has not been pursued as a treatment option in the modern era.

Attempting to reduce morbidity for treatment of prostate cancer, Flocks et al used visible application of a flat cryoprobe to the prostate and any obvious local extraglandular cancer extension through an open perineal surgical approach.[7] This approach avoided damage to the sphincter in this small series of 11 patients with minimal undefined complications reported. Although all patients had significant local cancer extension, no evidence of local recurrence was reported, most likely due to inconsistent and short duration of follow-up.

The first report of a transperineal percutaneous approach occurred in 1974 when Megalli et al used a single pointed 6.3 mm (18 Fr) liquid nitrogen cryoprobe introduced through a skin incision on either side of the perineal midline and guided its placement by digital palpation. Freezing was monitored digitally and often supplemented by a single thermostat in the peri-rectal region. The cryoprobe was typically repositioned one or more times to achieve adequate coverage of the prostate, seminal vesicles, and any palpably identifiable extraglandular extension.[8]

Subsequent investigators used visual and tactile control for insertion of a sharp cryoprobe in various modifications for both open and percutaneous transperineal access. Because cryogenic systems only had a single cryoprobe, several operators employed two units simultaneously to speed the process, repositioning the cryoprobes to achieve a large composite freezing effect.[9] Complications were frequent but judged to be less severe than those likely with conventional surgery, especially when applied to high-risk patients with advanced disease.[10] The cryosurgical mortality for prostate cancer treatment using these techniques was reported to be 1.9%.

Despite manipulation of the technique, however, it was apparent that cryotherapy was limited due to inability to place probes precisely and to adequately monitor the cryoablative process.[11] Cryotherapy was abandoned until the next major technical advances occurred in the early 1980s that led to development of a more controlled procedure with reduced morbidity.

DEVELOPMENT OF MODERN CRYOTHERAPY

Real-time image guidance and monitoring

The introduction and refinement of transrectal ultrasound (TRUS) was the critical technical component that afforded the opportunity for cryotherapy to be reconsidered as a modality for treatment of prostate cancer. TRUS provided a non-invasive method for both reliable assurance of probe placement within the prostate gland and an acoustical pattern that corresponded to ablative tissue changes. In the first of a series of seminal studies, Onik and colleagues described the characteristics of frozen prostate tissue in 1988.[12] They subsequently reported preliminary success with a significantly revised cryosurgical procedure characterized by three major innovations: real-time TRUS monitoring, multiple cryoprobes, and a urethral warming catheter.[12–14] These components remain the hallmark of current prostate cryotherapy.

Real-time ultrasound-guided placement of the cryoprobes and continuous visualization during freezing were the elements that first allowed physicians to encompass the entire gland with cryotherapy and still protect the rectum and other vital structures. Ice has an acoustic impedance much different than any tissue; it reflects up to 99% of the incident acoustic signal to create a well-delineated interface. Unfortunately, this strongly reflective interface is an impenetrable acoustic wall which renders everything behind the leading edge of approaching ice acoustically invisible. Thus sonography has limitations despite improved image quality and innovations such as duplex color Doppler imaging. This is exemplified with the curvilinear TRUS probes popularly used for TRUS-guided prostate biopsy which do not permit adequate visualization during the freezing process. The relatively small curvilinear face exaggerates loss of visualization during freezing with too much of the rectum unseen during the critical late stage of the procedure and use of this probe type may increase the risk of rectal injury.[15]

However, a biplanar ultrasound probe helps overcome this problem through the use of easily interchangeable crystals which allows monitoring of both cryoprobe placement and the approach of the ice interface toward the rectum (Figure 2.1). Unfortunately, bi-plane probes are not available from all manufacturers because of their limited utility in routine diagnostic work. Although color Doppler flow evaluation is not an objective parameter, addition of this measurement has been used by some cryosurgeons during treatment to provide some indication of the vascular state between the advancing ice interface (commonly known as the "iceball") and the rectal wall.

At this stage, information provided by the sonographic image is limited to anatomical localization and the presence of ice formation. Sonography provides no information about the temperature distribution within the ice nor does it show the extent of freezing at the lateral or anterior aspects of the prostate. Even experienced operators cannot reliably estimate the subzero temperature at the neurovascular bundles in the prostate by TRUS alone.[16] In addition, operators are biased that the tissue is colder than the actual temperature.[16] Reports from cryosurgeons who did not rely on visual images alone but used thermosensor monitoring during therapy claim objective improvement for their clinical results.[17,18] Others rely on frequent digital palpation of the prostate during the freeze to ensure that imaging artifact

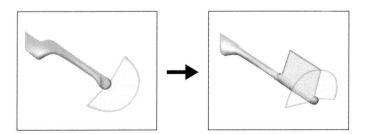

Figure 2.1 Biplanar transrectal ultrasound probe demonstrating bidimensional imaging pattern that allows visualization of probe placement and approaching ice formation.

does not cause misinterpretation of the freezing progression, an admittedly crude gauge of freeze extent at best.

Reports of three-dimensional (3-D) sonography during cryotherapy for preoperative planning and cryoprobe placement have potential to improve the procedure but clinical application is relatively laborious.[19] Furthermore, some of these techniques require fixation of the TRUS probe in a mechanical cradle that limits the ability to both manipulate the transducer and perform other tasks during the procedure. Advances in this technology are encouraging that rapid, practical 3-D imaging will be available in the future.

Both computed tomography (CT) and magnetic resonance imaging (MRI) can visualize the complete circumference of frozen tissue as well as demonstrate its internal structure.[14,20] CT guidance has proven feasible for real-time monitoring in phantom models, animal studies, and anecdotal human application.[21,22] The potential advantage of continuous real-time 3-D monitoring of the complete freeze progression by CT is negated due to imaging artifacts created by metal cryoprobes, the physical restriction of the gantry, and the continuous radiation exposure required. Likewise, CT cannot provide direct tissue temperature information by tissue density changes or other parameters.[23]

MR thermometry does have potential for real-time 3-D monitoring because it does not involve ionizing radiation while providing information about the entire tissue volume.[24,25] MR thermometry can correlate measurable MR signal with the actual temperature of frozen tissue down to the critical level of about $-40°C$.[24] Some of the open magnet scanner designs are more easily adapted to intra-operative use and may prove practical for clinical MR thermometry. However, MRI requires non-ferromagnetic operating instruments and patients with most pacemakers cannot undergo conventional MRI.

The only current potential utility of both MRI and CT imaging is in computer integration with mathematical models to generate real-time 3-D thermal maps of tissue freezing.[26–29] These models can create a volumetric thermal model of frozen tissue by integration of the visualized margin of freezing with temperature readings. The volumetric rendering can be fused with real-time images to create a virtual thermal map of the internal frozen prostate. However, the practical application of this technology awaits improvements in design to allow better access to the patient, higher resolution to adequately visualize the rectal wall, and lower cost in the current reimbursement climate.

Cryogenic technology

In addition to improvements in imaging, significant advances in cryoprobe technology stimulated a resurgence in clinical applications of cryotherapy. Early investigators used a single cryoprobe that had to be repositioned several times to create an overlap in the treatment field for successful tissue destruction (Figure 2.2). Tissue becomes visibly frozen between 0 and $-1°C$ but must be cooled to a much lower level (variably reported between $-20°C$ and $-50°C$) for reliable cancer cytotoxicity.[30] Only a small central volume of tissue reaches sufficiently cold temperatures for cancer eradication from a single cryoprobe. Repositioning of the single probe does not necessarily create an effectively larger treatment field because actual thermal distribution is unknown and the actual volume of tissue sufficiently frozen is underestimated.[15]

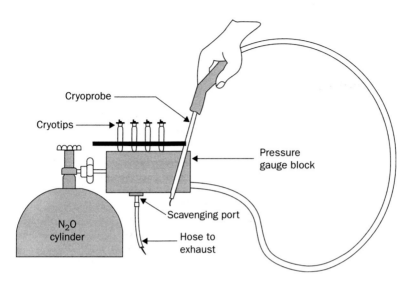

Figure 2.2 Illustration of an early liquid nitrogen cryosystem with large-diameter single probe.

However, multiple cryoprobes operated simultaneously achieve a synergistically uniform distribution of lethal temperature throughout the iceball.[28] Another advantage afforded by use of multiple probes is the ability to customize the shape of the ice formation to the contours of the individual prostate anatomy. One can vary the field of treatment through independent modulation of the individual probes which is now made possible with modern cryogenic technology. The type of cryogenic agent, the size and shape of probes, and variations in technique all modify the tissue distribution of the freeze and the cryogenic effect.

The first modern cryoprobe system was based on liquid nitrogen as a cryogen with independent throttle control of five cryoprobes (Accuprobe System, Cryomedical Sciences Inc., Rockville, MD, USA) that provided high-efficiency freezing.[14,31] This system was introduced in the early 1990s and featured several improvements over earlier liquid nitrogen systems. Refrigeration ("supercooling") of the liquid nitrogen to $-209°C$ from its usual boiling point at $-196°C$ eliminated problems with N_2 gas bubbles forming in the cryoprobes and their transport tubes. Gas bubbles form an insulating layer which can unpredictably impede liquid cryogen circulation. Furthermore, these new probes were vacuum insulated except for the distal few centimeters where the freeze effect occurs, thereby protecting tissues along the course of the cryoprobes from freezing. Interestingly, the iceball generated by these probes is an elongated ellipsoid that roughly corresponds to the anatomy of many prostate glands with a wider freeze zone at the base than the apex. Many of the early reports in the new era of cryotherapy were performed with this system.

Liquid nitrogen systems have limitations due to the inherent difficulties of control and circulation of the cryogenic agent. Reaction time to the operator changes during the procedure are relatively slow with this technology with a perceived delay of up to 2 minutes between command and response.[32] This can be problematic when the cryosurgeon desires to acutely reverse the freezing process. Maintenance of the system can be complex and require expertise not readily available within the standard

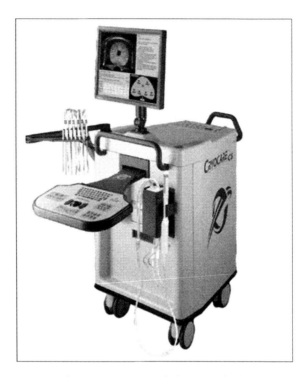

Figure 2.3   Latest version of argon gas system which uses multiple small-diameter cryoprobes with computerized dosimetry.

medical institution. Inconsistent cryoprobe performance may be due to accumulation of water or other contaminants within the conduction system.[15] In addition, the bulky liquid nitrogen system can limit operator access to the patient for probe placement.

Most cryotherapists use the more recently developed multiple port, high pressure gas systems (Endocare, Irvine CA, USA; Galil Medical, Yokneam, Israel) that utilize the Joule-Thompson (J-T) effect to create freezing (Figure 2.3). The J-T effect occurs when a gas under high pressure expands through a narrow port into a lower-pressure chamber. By circulating argon under high pressure (3000 psi), this constant expansion results in rapid cooling of argon gas to its boiling point (−186°C). The argon gas is circulated to the cryoprobe tip where it expands rapidly as it drops to room pressure (15 psi). The expanded gases are circulated back to the cryogenic unit through the larger outer lumen of the cryoprobe and the supply hose. Freezing is controlled by computer-modulated regulators that open and close the supply gas flow for each cryoprobe. The J-T effect is also used to reverse the freezing process rapidly for added effect in the freeze–thaw cycle. In this situation, helium becomes warmed under the J-T effect and is incorporated into the same system to act as a cryoprobe heater as it expands into a lower-pressure chamber. Used gas is vented at the cryogenic unit and care must be taken to have adequate air circulation in the treatment room to avoid oxygen displacement by these otherwise safe inert gases.

Gas systems are finely adjustable with rapid response to operator command, provide rapid conversion from freezing to heating, and are very compact for easy

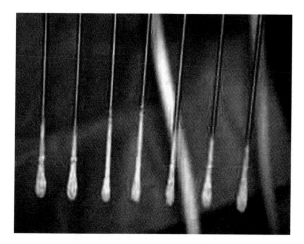

Figure 2.4 Small-diameter cryoprobes used simultaneously for treatment.

deployment in the operating theater. The argon system also creates an iceball more rapidly than liquid systems but both systems appear to have equal freezing capabilities after 10 minutes of treatment time.[15] The argon gas system can operate up to eight cryoprobes, providing more flexibility for customized freezing strategies, and is less prone to maintenance issues than its liquid nitrogen counterparts. Very-small-caliber probes are now available which create smaller iceballs but can be positioned without insertion kits (Figure 2.4); early reports demonstrate similar clinical complication rates but lack sufficient follow-up for conclusions of similar clinical efficacy in comparison to the larger-diameter probes.[33,34]

Urethral preservation

Another important advance in contemporary prostate cancer cryotherapy was the realization that maintenance of the urethral temperature above freezing minimized complications.[35-38] This is accomplished by placement of a urethral warming catheter during the freezing process. Although initially applied in the new era of prostate cryotherapy in the late 1980s, these systems were not uniform and their use was disallowed by the Food and Drug Administration (FDA) in the early 1990s. Alarmed by a rapid increase in complications reported by cryotherapy operators, the American Urological Association (AUA) collated data from nearly 1700 cryotherapy cases and compared complication rates with and without urethral warming catheters. The AUA demonstrated a significant increase in complication rates from 6% in cases with a urethral warmer to 24% in cases without the catheter. Furthermore, most of the increased complications were of a serious nature such as tissue sloughing with obstruction, hematuria requiring intervention, incontinence, and need for secondary procedures. Most troubling was the rise in rectal perforation rates from less than 2% to 7%. Armed with those data, the AUA successfully petitioned the FDA for an immediate reversal of the ban on urethral warming catheters.

This double-lumen catheter is commercially available and is now considered an important integral component of the procedure. A pump and warmer circulates a saline solution which preserves a thin layer of mucosa and underlying tissue visible on both subsequent MRI and histological evaluation.[39,40] Contemporary reports demonstrate a return to significantly decreased complication rates with the warmer, including an acceptable rectal perforation rate of 1% or less.[17,18,31,36,41–44]

FUTURE OF CRYOTHERAPY

Cryotherapy clearly has a role in the management of localized prostate cancer and is currently the only viable therapeutic option for radiation failures other than surgery.[45,46] Continued refinement of the techniques, delivery mechanisms, and imaging will continue to advance this modality. Computer simulation is being used for prediction of treatment fields and treatment planning for customized optimal probe placement.[47] Virtual reality surgical simulation with haptic feedback has been used to develop training modules for aspiring cryotherapists.[48]

The shifting paradigm for prostate cancer has opened another potential avenue for cryotherapy of localized prostate cancer. Whereas prostate cancer dogma in the past dictated multifocality at time of presentation, the changes in detection rates toward lower-stage, lower-grade cancers in younger men have now led to a significant cohort of patients with relatively smaller-volume prostate cancer.

With more men interested in the possibility of minimally invasive approaches to avoid the complication rates of surgery and external beam radiation, the potential for focal treatment of prostate cancer by cryotherapy is being explored.[49] Data from radiologic series demonstrate significantly improved biochemical disease-free rates following brachytherapy with seed placement guided and modified by local signal intensity distribution within the prostate found on ProstaScint scans (capromab pendetide, Cytogen Corporation, Princeton, NJ, USA) (Figure 2.5).[50] This localization is made possible by the dramatic improvements in resolution afforded by dual-head gamma scanners with fusion of ProstaScint images to CT.[51,52] The 7-year follow-up data

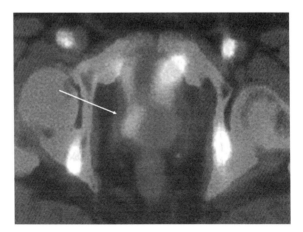

Figure 2.5 Computed tomography and SPECT scan (ProstaScint) fused image demonstrating increased signal in the prostate right peripheral zone (arrow). Seven-year brachytherapy outcomes data with treatment guided by fused scans support the use of cryotherapy for focal treatment of localized prostate cancer in selected cases.

recently reported on 239 patients demonstrated significantly improved biochemical disease-free recurrence outcomes in patients across all risk stratification classes compared to the 5-year meta-analysis of brachytherapy (96% vs 87% low risk, 87% vs 74% intermediate risk, 73% vs 50% high risk).[53,54] Extrapolation from these data for localized cryotherapy is reasonable and currently being pursued. It is believed that focal cryotherapy will avoid some of the undesirable outcomes, such as relatively high erectile dysfunction rates, historically associated with prostate cryotherapy.

The evolutionary process for prostate cryotherapy has been circuitous and dependent upon technological advances and greater understanding of the effect of freezing on tumor biology in a controlled fashion. Advances of imaging technology, computational power, and delivery mechanisms will continue to refine this process and ensure that cryotherapy remains a viable option for treatment of localized disease.

REFERENCES

1. Gage AA. History of cryosurgery. Semin Surg Oncol 1998; 14: 99–109.
2. Rubinsky B. Cryosurgery. Annu Rev Biomed Eng 2000; 2: 157–87.
3. Gage AA. Cryosurgery in the treatment of cancer. Surg Gynecol Obstet 1992; 174: 73–92.
4. Cooper I, Lee A. Cryostatic congelation: a system for producing a limited controlled region of cooling or freezing of biological tissue. J Nerv Ment Dis 1961; 133: 259–6.
5. Gonder MJ, Soanes WA, Shulman S. Cryosurgical treatment of the prostate. Invest Urol 1966; 3: 372–8.
6. Soanes WA, Gonder MJ. Use of cryosurgery in prostatic cancer. J Urol 1968; 99: 793–7.
7. Flocks RH, Nelson CM, Boatman DL. Perineal cryosurgery for prostatic carcinoma. J Urol 1972; 108: 933–5.
8. Megalli MR, Gursel EO, Veenema RJ. Closed perineal cryosurgery in prostatic cancer. New probe and technique. Urology 1974; 4: 220–2.
9. Kunit G. "Open perineal cryosurgery" in carcinoma of the prostate – a possible curative alternative. Urol Res 1986; 14: 3–7.
10. Loening S, Hawtrey C, Bonney W et al. Perineal cryosurgery of prostate cancer. Urology 1981; 17: 12–14.
11. Bonney WW, Fallon B, Gerber WL et al. Cryosurgery in prostatic cancer: survival. Urology 1982; 19: 37–42.
12. Onik G, Cobb C, Cohen J, Zabkar J, Porterfield B. US characteristics of frozen prostate. Radiology 1988; 168: 629–31.
13. Rubinsky B, Gilbert JC, Onik GM et al. Monitoring cryosurgery in the brain and in the prostate with proton NMR. Cryobiology 1993; 30: 191–9.
14. Onik GM, Cohen JK, Reyes GD et al. Transrectal ultrasound-guided percutaneous radical cryosurgical ablation of the prostate. Cancer 1993; 72: 1291–9.
15. Saliken JC, Donnelly BJ, Rewcastle J. The evolution and state of modern technology for prostate cryosurgery. Urology 2002; 60: 26–33.
16. Steed J, Saliken J, Donnelly BJ, Ali-Ridha NH. Correlation between thermosensor temperature and transrectal ultrasonography during prostate cryoablation. Can Assoc Radiol J 1997; 48: 186–90.
17. Lee F, Bahn DK, Badalament RA et al. Cryosurgery for prostate cancer: improved glandular ablation by use of 6 to 8 cryoprobes. Urology 1999; 54: 135–40.
18. Wong WS, Chinn DO, Chinn M et al. Cryosurgery as a treatment for prostate carcinoma: results and complications. Cancer 1997; 79: 963–74.
19. Chin JL, Downey DB, Mulligan M, Fenster A. Three-dimensional transrectal ultrasound guided cryoablation for localized prostate cancer in nonsurgical candidates: a feasibility study and report of early results. J Urol 1998; 159: 910–14.

20. Isoda H. [Sequential MRI and CT monitoring in cryosurgery – an experimental study in rats]. Nippon Igaku Hoshasen Gakkai Zasshi 1989; 49: 1499–508.
21. Lee FT Jr, Chosy SG, Littrup PJ et al. CT-monitored percutaneous cryoablation in a pig liver model: pilot study. Radiology 1999; 211: 687–92.
22. Saliken JC, McKinnon JG, Gray R. CT for monitoring cryotherapy. AJR Am J Roentgenol 1996; 166: 853–5.
23. Sandison GA, Loye MP, Rewcastle JC et al. X-ray CT monitoring of iceball growth and thermal distribution during cryosurgery. Phys Med Biol 1998; 43: 3309–24.
24. Wansapura JP, Daniel BL, Pauly J, Butts K. Temperature mapping of frozen tissue using eddy current compensated half excitation RF pulses. Magn Reson Med 2001; 46: 985–92.
25. Daniel BL, Butts K, Block WF. Magnetic resonance imaging of frozen tissues: temperature-dependent MR signal characteristics and relevance for MR monitoring of cryosurgery. Magn Reson Med 1999; 41: 627–30.
26. Gilbert JC, Rubinsky B, Wong ST et al. Temperature determination in the frozen region during cryosurgery of rabbit liver using MR image analysis. Magn Reson Imaging 1997; 15: 657–67.
27. Rewcastle JC, Sandison GA, Hahn LJ et al. A model for the time-dependent thermal distribution within an iceball surrounding a cryoprobe. Phys Med Biol 1998; 43: 3519–34.
28. Jankun M, Kelly TJ, Zaim A et al. Computer model for cryosurgery of the prostate. Comput Aided Surg 1999; 4: 193–9.
29. Gage AA, Baust J. Mechanisms of tissue injury in cryosurgery. Cryobiology 1998; 37: 171–86.
30. Chang Z, Finkelstein JJ, Ma H, Baust J. Development of a high-performance multiprobe cryosurgical device. Biomed Instrum Technol 1994; 28: 383–90.
31. Saliken JC, Donnelly BJ, Ernst S et al. Prostate cryotherapy: practicalities and applications from the Calgary experience. Can Assoc Radiol J 2001; 52: 165–73.
32. Rewcastle JC, Sandison GA, Saliken JC et al. Considerations during clinical operation of two commercially available cryomachines. J Surg Oncol 1999; 71: 106–11.
33. Leibovici D, Zisman A, Siegel YI, Lindner A. Cryosurgical ablation for prostate cancer: preliminary results of a new advanced technique. Isr Med Assoc 2001; 3: 484–7.
34. Gould RS. Total cryosurgery of the prostate versus standard cryosurgery versus radical prostatectomy: comparison of early results and the role of transurethral resection in cryosurgery. J Urol 1999; 162: 1653–7.
35. Cespedes RD, Pisters LL, von Eschenbach AC, McGuire EJ. Long-term followup of incontinence and obstruction after salvage cryosurgical ablation of the prostate: results in 143 patients. J Urol 1997; 157: 237–40.
36. Long JP, Bahn D, Lee F et al. Five-year retrospective, multi-institutional pooled analysis of cancer-related outcomes after cryosurgical ablation of the prostate. Urology 2001; 57: 518–23.
37. Cox RL, Crawford ED. Complications of cryosurgical ablation of the prostate to treat localized adenocarcinoma of the prostate. Urology 1995; 45: 932–5.
38. Vellet AD, Saliken J, Donnelly B et al. Prostatic cryosurgery: use of MR imaging in evaluation of success and technical modifications. Radiology 1997; 203: 653–9.
39. Donnelly BJ, Saliken JC, Ali-Ridha N et al. Histological findings in the prostate two years following cryosurgical ablation. Can J Urol 2001; 8: 1237–9.
40. Milsten R. Urethral warmer survey. Urology 1995; 45: 171.
41. Saliken JC, Donnelly BJ, Brasher P et al. Outcome and safety of transrectal US-guided percutaneous cryotherapy for localized prostate cancer. J Vasc Interv Radiol 1999; 10: 199–208.
42. Ellis DE. Cryosurgery as a primary treatment for localized prostate cancer: a community hospital experience. Urology 2002; 60: 34–9.
43. Shinohara K. Prostate cancer: cryotherapy. Urol Clin North Am 2003; 30(4): 725–36.
44. Johnson DB, Nakada SY. Cryoablation of renal and prostate tumors. J Endourol 2003; 17: 627–32.
45. Izawa JI, Madsen LT, Scott SM et al. Salvage cryotherapy for recurrent prostate cancer after radiotherapy: variables affecting patient outcome. J Clin Oncol 2002; 20: 2664–71.

46. Touma NJ, Izawa JI, Chin JL. Current status of local salvage therapies following radiation failure for prostate cancer. J Urol 2005; 173: 373–9.
47 Rewcastle JC, Sandison GA, Muldrew K et al. A model for the time dependent three-dimensional thermal distribution within iceballs surrounding multiple cryoprobes. Med Phys 2001; 28: 1125–37.
48. Hahn JK, Manyak MJ, Jin G et al. Cryotherapy simulator for localized prostate cancer. Stud Health Technol Inform 2002; 85: 173–8.
49. Onik G. The male lumpectomy: rationale for a cancer targeted approach for prostate cryoablation. A review. Technol Cancer Res Treat 2004; 3: 365–70.
50. Ellis RJ, Vertocnik A, Kim E et al. Four-year biochemical outcome after radioimmuno-guided transperineal brachytherapy for patients with prostate adenocarcinoma. Int J Radiat Oncol Biol Phys 2003; 57: 362–70.
51. Schettino CJ, Kramer EL, Noz ME et al. Impact of fusion of indium-111 capromab pendetide volume data sets with those from MRI or CT in patients with recurrent prostate cancer. AJR Am J Roentgenol 2004; 183: 519–24.
52. Sodee DB, Nelson AD, Faulhaber PF et al. Update on fused capromab pendetide imaging of prostate cancer. Clin Prostate Cancer 2005; 3: 230–8.
53. Ellis RJ, Kim E, Zhou H et al. Seven-year biochemical disease-free survival rates following permanent prostate brachytherapy with dose escalation to biological tumor volumes (BTVs) identified with SPECT/CT image fusion. Abstract #121, American Brachytherapy Society, 2005.
54. Quaranta BP, Marks LB, Anscher MS. Comparing radical prostatectomy and brachytherapy for localized prostate cancer. Oncology 2004; 18: 1289–302.

3

Pathologic findings after prostatic cryoablation

Isabelle Meiers, David G. Bostwick

Introduction • **Mechanisms of tissue cryoablation** • **Findings: histopathologic**
• **Conclusion**

INTRODUCTION

Cryotherapy is an effective treatment for select prostate lesions, creating reproducible and predictable pathologic changes in tissue.[1-6] This report briefly summa-
rizes current understanding of the mechanisms of cryoablation and the pathologic
findings in the prostate.

MECHANISMS OF TISSUE CRYOABLATION

Cryosurgery relies on rapid freezing, slow thawing, and repetition of the freeze–thaw
cycle. As the temperature drops, extracellular water crystallizes and forms a hyperosmotic extracellular environment that draws water out of the cell. Extracellular ice
crystals grow and compress the dehydrating cell membranes, resulting in severe
damage. This effect of cell dehydration and solution concentration is called solution-
effect injury. Up to this point, the damage is reversible. The process is irreversible
when there is intracellular ice formation; this is usually associated with rapid freezing
(several degrees centigrade per minute). Pure water begins to freeze at 0°C, and extracellular ice forms at approximately −8°C; by −15°C, intracellular ice begins to form,
and, by −50°C, all metabolic processes cease. Faster freezing rates and lower end temperatures have the most deleterious effects on tissue. The cooling rate should be as
fast as possible, but the thawing rate, and the coldest tissue temperature reached are
the principal destructive factors, and thawing should be as slow as possible. Repetition of the freeze–thaw cycle is important for effective therapy.[7] Cryosurgery kills cells
and destroys tissue by mechanisms that feature direct cell injury from ice crystal
formation and related deleterious effects and vascular stasis caused by microcirculatory failure.[8] Recently a third mechanism of cell death associated with cryosurgery has
been identified. This mechanism, apoptosis or gene-regulated cell death, is additive
with the direct ice-related cell damage that occurs during the operative freeze–thaw
intervals and coagulative necrosis that occurs in the following days post-treatment.[9,10]

FINDINGS: HISTOPATHOLOGIC

Histopathologic results are considered by most to be the best absolute method for
determining the extent of ablation within the prostate. Cryosurgical ablation results in

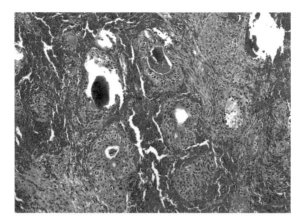

Figure 3.1 Stromal hemorrhage with residual viable epithelium following prostatic cryoablation (×100 magnification). (See also color plate.)

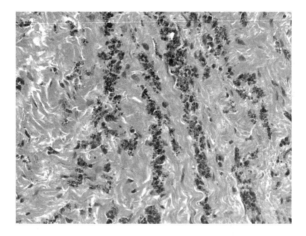

Figure 3.2 Hemosiderin deposition (ochre pigment) within the stroma after cryosurgery (×400 magnification). (See also color plate.)

substantial tissue destruction of benign and malignant cells and there appear to be little or no differential effects on epithelium or stroma; virtually all tissue contained within the ablative zone is destroyed. Following cryosurgery, the thin rim of viable surviving tissue of the prostate shows typical features of repair, including marked stromal fibrosis and hyalinization, basal cell hyperplasia with ductal and acinar regeneration, squamous metaplasia, urothelial metaplasia, stromal hemorrhage (Figure 3.1) and hemosiderin deposition (Figure 3.2).[11–15] Coagulative necrosis with devitalization is observed up to 30 weeks after therapy (Figure 3.3), but patchy chronic inflammation is more common in the late stages (Figure 3.4). The radius of necrosis was 6.0 mm around a single cryoprobe after a double freeze. An array of cryprobes must be placed in the prostate to create adequate temperatures to ablate large areas of tissue. It is crucial to measure temperatures by thermocouple at the periphery and within the

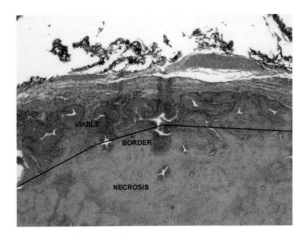

Figure 3.3 Coagulative necrosis (bottom of image) with devitalization and a thin rim of sub-capsular viable tissue (top) following cryosurgery; dog prostate (×100 magnification). (See also color plate.)

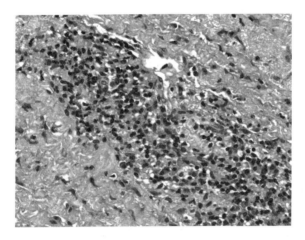

Figure 3.4 Patchy chronic inflammation within prostatic stroma is a common finding following cryoablation (×400 magnification). (See also color plate.)

prostate to ensure adequate ablation. Tissue damage extends about 1.5 mm beyond the edge of the necrosis, and is characterized by squamous metaplasia and hemorrhage, as reported in patients who underwent initial cryosurgery followed by radical retropubic prostatectomy 2–3 weeks later.[16] Focal granulomatous inflammation may also occur with epithelial disruption due to corpora amylacea. Dystrophic calcification is infrequent, and usually appears in areas with the greatest reparative response.

After cryosurgery, are malignant and benign components within the prostate gland totally ablated? To date, few studies have assessed the long-term pathologic findings after cryoablation. Atypia and high-grade prostatic intraepithelial neoplasia are not seen in areas that otherwise show changes of post-cryoablation therapy. Biopsy after cryosurgery may reveal no evidence of recurrent or residual carcinoma, even in some patients with elevated prostate-specific antigen (PSA). Some investigators reported residual malignant cells in 7–23% of men with areas of viable benign glands in 45–70% of patients.[17] In two other studies, positive biopsy findings were reported in 13% and 18% of patients after cryosurgery with or without androgen deprivation therapy.[18,19] Recently, some authors reported persistence of cancer cells in the 6- and 12-month biopsies in 11% and 5.5%, respectively; all 24-month biopsies were negative,[20] suggesting continued destruction over time, similar to radiation therapy. Other authors reported their experience with high-risk patients (defined as either a PSA level ≥ 10 ng/ml, or a Gleason sum score ≥ 8, or both) who were unwilling to undergo radical surgery or radiation therapy. On postcryosurgery biopsies 12.5% were positive.[21] No patient had progressed at last follow-up, and the overall survival rate was 100%.[21] The results for a series of 176 patients who underwent cryosurgery for clinically localized disease were reported by Koppie et al 57% of patients had neoadjuvant androgen deprivation. The cancer stage was T1 in 8.7%, T2 in 30%, T3 in 59% and T4 in 2.3%. The nadir PSA level was undetectable in 49% of patients, 0.1–0.4 in 21% and > 0.5 ng/ml in 30% after cryosurgery. After 43% of procedures, the serum PSA reached a nadir of < 0.5 ng/ml and did not increase by > 0.2 ng/ml on at least two occasions. However, prostate biopsies were positive after 38% of procedures.[22]

In some cases, the benign prostate and cancer appear unchanged, with no change in grade (Figure 3.5) or definite evidence of tissue or immune response; indicating lack of inclusion of that area in the ablation killing zone. As the postoperative interval increases, biopsy is more likely to contain unaltered benign prostatic tissue. Bahn et al investigated the relationship between DNA ploidy and the efficacy of cryoablation and demonstrated that outcome is independent of DNA ploidy status.[24] There is no consensus regarding grading after cryoablation therapy, and most pathologists (including us) routinely report Gleason grade.

Cryotherapy of the prostate represents a potential treatment for localized recurrent prostate cancer after radiation therapy, and several studies have reported salvage

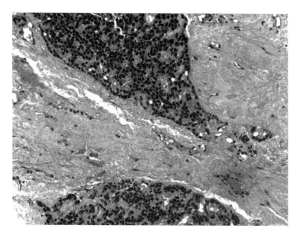

Figure 3.5   Residual/recurrent adenocarcinoma (Gleason 4 + 4 = 8) indicating lack of treatment effect; tumor appeared unchanged, with no change in grade or definite evidence of tissue or immune response (×200 magnification). (See also color plate.)

cryotherapy results after biopsy-proven local failure after external beam radiotherapy.[25-35] The most worrisome finding is with the postcryotherapy histopathologic evaluation; the presence of residual or recurrent cancer is considered evidence of inadequate cryotherapy and inadequate radiotherapy. In one study of patients with biopsy-proven local failure after external beam radiotherapy, the combination of neoadjuvant androgen deprivation therapy with salvage cryotherapy reported residual cancer, viable benign prostate glands, and viable stroma in 14%, 42%, and 27%, respectively.[26] These biopsy results were obtained with four-core sampling and therefore likely underestimated the true incidence of residual cancer.[26] A cohort of 59 patients who had been previously treated with radiation therapy and had rising serum PSA values underwent salvage cryoablation of the prostate for localized, histologically proven, recurrent prostate cancer.[35] No biopsies (0%) showed evidence of residual or recurrent disease.[35]

The MD Anderson Cancer Center experience reported positive biopsy specimens in 17% of patients after salvage cryotherapy for recurrent prostate cancer after biopsy-proven external beam radiotherapy failure.[27] Another study reported that the presence of cancer cells in the biopsy was the only histopathologic variable that adversely affected disease-free survival; the finding of atypical or normal epithelial tissue in biopsy specimens after salvage cryotherapy was not predictive of biochemical failure.[28] Lee et al reported a local control rate of 65% with salvage cryotherapy following radiation failure.[32]

No definitive method exists for assessment of tumor viability after cryoablation. PSA and PAP expression persists in benign and malignant epithelium, suggesting that tumor cells capable of protein production probably retain the potential for cell division and consequent metastatic spread. Keratin 34βE12, p63 (both basal cell-specific markers) and racemase expression also persist after cryoablation (Figures 3.6A,B), and are of diagnostic value in separating treated adenocarcinoma and its mimics.

There is a strong correlation between magnetic resonance imaging (MRI) with gadolinium defects and amount of coagulation necrosis caused within the prostate by minimally invasive techniques.[36] Difficulty arises in the evaluation of cryosurgical ablation patients because of the damage zone created by the treatment.[16]

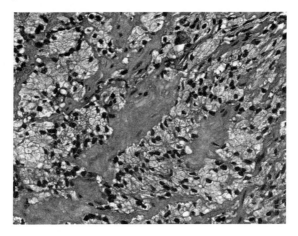

Figure 3.6A   Residual/recurrent adenocarcinoma (Gleason 4 + 3 = 7) (400× magnification). (See also color plate.)

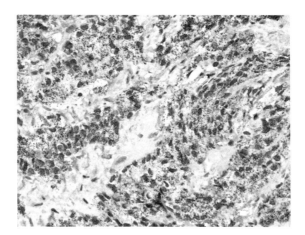

Figure 3.6B   Intense racemase stain in cancer. There is prominent immunoreactivity (granular red reaction product) in most of the secretory cells. There is no immunoreactivity (absence of brown reaction product) for basal cell-specific high-molecular-weight keratin (34βE12) and p63 (400× magnification). (See also color plate.)

However, gadolinium defects were not seen in areas of viable tissue as determined by histopathologic evaluation.[36] However, some investigators reported that findings of postoperative gadolinium-enhanced MRI were not predictive of 6-month biopsy results or follow-up PSA levels.[37]

CONCLUSION

Cryotherapy effectively and reproducibly ablates benign and neoplastic epithelium and stroma in the prostate, with consistent histopathologic findings that include central coagulative necrosis surrounded by a thin rim of tissue displaying reparative changes.

REFERENCES

1. American Cancer Society. Cancer Facts and Figures. Atlanta, GA: American Cancer Society, 2006: 4. www.cancer.org.
2. Anastasiadis AG, Sachdev R, Salomon L et al. Comparison of health-related quality of life and prostate-associated symptoms after primary and salvage cryotherapy for prostate cancer. J Cancer Res Clin Oncol 2003; 129 (12): 676–82.
3. Onik G. The male lumpectomy: rationale for a cancer targeted approach for prostate cryoablation. A review. Technol Cancer Res Treat 2004; 3 (4): 365–70.
4. Merrick GS, Wallner KE, Butler WM. Prostate cryotherapy: more questions than answers. Urology 2005; 66 (1): 9–15.
5. Pareek G, Nakada SY. The current role of cryotherapy for renal and prostate tumors. Urol Oncol 2005; 23 (5): 361–6.
6. Vestal JC. Critical review of the efficacy and safety of cryotherapy of the prostate. Curr Urol Rep 2005; 6 (3): 190–3.
7. Gage AA, Baust J. Mechanisms of tissue injury in cryosurgery. Cryobiology 1998; 37 (3): 171–86.

8. Baust JG, Gage AA. The molecular basis of cryosurgery. BJU Int 2005; 95 (9): 1187–91.
9. Gage AA, Baust JG. Cryosurgery – a review of recent advances and current issues. Cryo Letters 2002; 23 (2): 69–78.
10. Baust JG, Gage AA, Clarke D et al. Cryosurgery – a putative approach to molecular-based optimization. Cryobiology 2004; 48 (2): 190–204.
11. Petersen DS, Milleman LA, Rose EF et al. Biopsy and clinical course after cryosurgery for prostatic cancer. J Urol 1978; 120 (3): 308–11.
12. Shabaik A, Wilson S, Bidair M et al. Pathologic changes in prostate biopsies following cryoablation therapy of prostate carcinoma. J Urol Pathol 1995; 3: 183–94.
13. Borkowski P, Robinson MJ, Poppiti RJ Jr, Nash SC. Histologic findings in postcryosurgical prostatic biopsies. Mod Pathol 1996; 9 (8): 807–11.
14. Falconieri G, Lugnani F, Zanconati F et al. Histopathology of the frozen prostate. The microscopic bases of prostatic carcinoma cryoablation. Pathol Res Pract 1996; 192 (6): 579–87.
15. Shuman BA, Cohen JK, Miller RJ Jr et al. Histological presence of viable prostatic glands on routine biopsy following cryosurgical ablation of the prostate. J Urol 1997; 157 (2): 552–5.
16. Larson TR, Robertson DW, Corica A, Bostwick DG. In vivo interstitial temperature mapping of the human prostate during cryosurgery with correlation to histopathologic outcomes. Urology 2000; 55 (4): 547–52.
17. Shinohara K. Prostate cancer: cryotherapy. Urol Clin North Am 2003; 30 (4): 725–36.
18. Bahn DK, Lee F, Badalament R et al. Targeted cryoablation of the prostate: 7-year outcomes in the primary treatment of prostate cancer. Urology 2002; 60 (2 Suppl 1): 3–11.
19. Long JP, Bahn D, Lee F, Shinohara K et al. Five-year retrospective, multi-institutional pooled analysis of cancer-related outcomes after cryosurgical ablation of the prostate. Urology 2001; 57 (3): 518–23.
20. Escudero Barrilero A, Arias Funez F, Rodriguez-Patron Rodriguez R, Garcia Gonzalez R. [Cryotherapy III, bibligraphic review. Our experience(II)]. Arch Esp Urol 2005; 58 (10): 1003–29.
21. Prepelica KL, Okeke Z, Murphy A, Katz AE. Cryosurgical ablation of the prostate: high risk patient outcomes. Cancer 2005; 103 (8): 1625–30.
22. Koppie TM, Shinohara K, Grossfeld GD et al. The efficacy of cryosurgical ablation of prostate cancer: the University of California, San Francisco experience. J Urol 1999; 162 (2): 427–32.
23. Pisters LL, Dinney CP, Pettaway CA et al. A feasibility study of cryotherapy followed by radical prostatectomy for locally advanced prostate cancer. J Urol 1999; 161 (2): 509–14.
24. Bahn DK, Silverman P, Lee F Sr et al. In treating localized prostate cancer the efficacy of cryoablation is independent of DNA ploidy type. Technol Cancer Res Treat 2004; 3 (3): 253–7.
25. Donnelly BJ, Saliken JC, Ernst DS et al. Role of transrectal ultrasound guided salvage cryosurgery for recurrent prostate carcinoma after radiotherapy. Prostate Cancer Prostatic Dis 2005; 8 (3): 235–42.
26. Chin JL, Touma N, Pautler SE et al. Serial histopathology results of salvage cryoablation for prostate cancer after radiation failure. J Urol 2003; 170 (4 Pt 1): 1199–202.
27. Izawa JI, Madsen LT, Scott SM et al. Salvage cryotherapy for recurrent prostate cancer after radiotherapy: variables affecting patient outcome. J Clin Oncol 2002; 20 (11): 2664–71.
28. Izawa JI, Morganstern N, Chan DM et al. Incomplete glandular ablation after salvage cryotherapy for recurrent prostate cancer after radiotherapy. Int J Radiat Oncol Biol Phys 2003; 56 (2): 468–72.
29. Chin JL, Touma N. Current status of salvage cryoablation for prostate cancer following radiation failure. Technol Cancer Res Treat 2005; 4 (2): 211–16.
30. Touma NJ, Izawa JI, Chin JL. Current status of local salvage therapies following radiation failure for prostate cancer. J Urol 2005; 173 (2): 373–9.
31. Ahmed S, Lindsey B, Davies J. Salvage cryosurgery for locally recurrent prostate cancer following radiotherapy. Prostate Cancer Prostatic Dis 2005; 8 (1): 31–5.

32. Lee F, Bahn DK, McHugh TA et al. Cryosurgery of prostate cancer. Use of adjuvant hormonal therapy and temperature monitoring – A one year follow-up. Anticancer Res 1997; 17 (3A): 1511–15.
33. Pisters LL, Perrotte P, Scott SM et al. Patient selection for salvage cryotherapy for locally recurrent prostate cancer after radiation therapy. J Clin Oncol 999; 17 (8): 2514–20.
34. de la Taille A, Hayek O, Benson MC et al. Salvage cryotherapy for recurrent prostate cancer after radiation therapy: the Columbia experience. Urology 2000; 55 (1): 79–84.
35. Bahn DK, Lee F, Silverman P et al. Salvage cryosurgery for recurrent prostate cancer after radiation therapy: a seven-year follow-up. Clin Prostate Cancer 2003; 2 (2): 111–14.
36. Larson BT, Collins JM, Huidobro C et al. Gadolinium-enhanced MRI in the evaluation of minimally invasive treatments of the prostate: correlation with histopathologic findings. Urology 2003; 62 (5): 900–4.
37. Donnelly SE, Donnelly BJ, Saliken JC et al. Prostate cancer: gadolinium-enhanced MR imaging at 3 weeks compared with needle biopsy at 6 months after cryoablation. Radiology 2004; 232 (3): 830–3.

4

Prostate cryosurgery

Ralph J. Miller Jr, Jeffrey K. Cohen

Introduction • Background and history • Indications • Technique • Results
• Interpretation of cryosurgery results • Complications

INTRODUCTION

Prostate cryosurgery is unique among the currently available potentially curative treatments for clinically localized prostate cancer. It is minimally invasive in a way similar to prostate brachytherapy, but without the use of radiation. Under ideal circumstances, it has an essentially ablative result, but without an incision. While prostate cryosurgery has a wide potential application, it has shown particular promise in the management of prostate cancer patients whose features don't fit neatly into the desirable criteria for the other therapies, for example high-risk disease and radiation failure. Prostate cryosurgery can be a valuable tool in the treatment armamentarium of the urologist who is well versed in its use.

BACKGROUND AND HISTORY

Therapeutic uses of cold temperatures applied to human body tissues date back to antiquity. Antineoplastic uses of cold temperatures date back at least 100 years. The first application of cold thermal energy to the prostate is credited to Gonder and Soanes who performed transurethral prostate cryosurgery in 1964. They used a transurethrally placed Van Buren sound-like cryoprobe positioned in the prostatic urethra. This freezing of the prostatic urethra and periurethral prostate tissue was used as a substitute for TURP in certain high-risk patients. While application of cold temperatures in this way did ablate periprostatic tissue, it also produced a problem that would become a recurring theme in the development of prostate cryosurgery, i.e. the sloughing of necrotic prostate tissue into the urinary stream. This "sloughing" produces a syndrome of undesirable side effects and sometimes requires additional procedures for management.

The use of cryosurgery specifically for prostate cancer was developed by Drs. Bonney, Loening, Schmidt et al at the University of Iowa in the 1970s. Many of the patients treated in this series had locally advanced prostate cancer and were not good candidates for surgical removal at the time. An open transperineal approach was utilized. The prostate was frozen under visual guidance by serially applying a hand-held cryoprobe to the surface of the exposed prostate until it had been completely frozen by visual assessment. Subsequent follow-up studies of the 200+ patients treated in this manner seemed to show significant antineoplastic effect at 10 years follow-up, but a subsequent re-review by Porter et al cast doubt on this earlier assessment. Still present were the issues of postoperative sloughing, as well as a newer problem with the development of fistulous tracts from prostate to skin or prostate to rectum in some patients.

Percutaneous transperineal prostate cryosurgery, essentially as it is performed today, was developed in the early 1990s by Cohen and Onik. Several available technologies were combined to produce a procedure that was minimally invasive and which could completely ablate the prostate. Three-millimeter diameter cylindrical cryoprobes were placed transperineally into the prostate in a series of steps beginning with needle placement and progressing to Amplatz-like dilators and finally to cryoprobes in direct apposition to the tissue in question. The probe insertion, positioning, and freezing steps were all monitored real time with transrectal ultrasound imaging of the prostate and periprostatic tissues. Control and monitoring of the process was made possible primarily by the dramatic change in the ultrasound appearance of tissue as it froze. With this enhanced control of the freezing process, and the addition of thermal protection of the prostatic urethra during the freezing process, the procedure as developed by Cohen and Onik addressed past concerns of both completeness and of excessively high morbidity encountered in earlier series. Further refinements in available equipment and surgical technique over the ensuing 15 years have enhanced the original procedure and have refined the results. Cryosurgical equipment has evolved from liquid nitrogen-based technology with the aforementioned 3-mm diameter cryoprobes to machines using high-pressure argon gas and the Jewell-Thompson effect to produce cooling. Probe size has been miniaturized down to a current 1.7-mm diameter making "cryoprobes" into "cryoneedles" with the attendant reduction in tissue trauma. Using cryoneedles allows prostate cryosurgery to be performed in a way completely similar to prostate brachytherapy. This has had a favorable impact on the learning curve associated with prostate cryosurgery.

INDICATIONS

The first 383 patients treated with prostate cryosurgery at our institution were treated on an IRB-approved protocol. Inclusion criteria were broad and included patients with T1–T3 disease, with any Gleason grade and any pre-treatment PSA. During and since that time, however, prostate cryosurgery has fit into a larger institutional philosophy of treatment selection for men with newly diagnosed prostate cancer. That philosophy places a heavy emphasis on patient education and patient participation in the decision-making process. Emphasis is also placed on choosing a therapy well suited to the patient's presenting scenerio according to the strengths and weaknesses of all of the treatment options available. For instance, a 55-year-old healthy man with T1 disease would be educated about cryosurgery, external beam radiation, and brachytherapy, but ultimately would be steered toward the traditional approach of radical prostatectomy as being the "first pick" to consider in his situation. As we gained experience with prostate cryosurgery in many clinical scenerios over the first several years of the protocol, it became clear that cryosurgery had some advantages in certain patient subsets compared with the other modalities. For instance, in our hands, cryosurgery has been a better option than salvage prostatectomy for well-selected patients with early failure following external beam radiation or brachytherapy. Inclusion criteria for this group includes a rising post-radiation PSA, positive post-radiation prostate needle biopsies, and a negative metastatic survey. At least three consecutive PSA rises following nadir (RTOG definition), and a positive biopsy at a minimum of 18 months post-radiation are required. "Early-failure" patients tend to fare the best, meaning patients whose PSA is still less than 10 and patients who have not already failed hormonal therapy. Another patient subset for which we have used cryosurgery extensively is patients with high-risk features. Patients who have one or more of the following – high-grade disease (Gleason 7 or higher), high PSA (greater than 10 ng/ml), or high-volume (multiple cores with high percentage involvement) disease – all have a lower rate of cure with the radiation options than do low-risk patients. Prostate cryosurgery is able to achieve local control in the great majority of these patients with minimal morbidity. Especially in older patients with high-risk prostate cancer, cryosurgery may be the best choice among the options. For example, a 72-year-old patient with a large-volume Gleason 7 tumor in several cores and a PSA of 15 may not be a good candidate for watchful waiting. He certainly could be treated with external beam therapy, brachytherapy, androgen deprivation therapy, or a combination of therapies, but his failure rate would be fairly high and salvage therapy would be more complicated. Long-term morbidity with radiation is considerable as well. Using cryosurgery monotherapy as an initial treatment strategy for this type of patient will often yield favorable results without altering future treatment options.

A wide variety of other specific situations can be treated with cryosurgery as well. Morbidly obese patients who are not candidates for radical prostatectomy or external beam radiation have been successfully treated with cryosurgery. Patients who have had rectal radiation for rectal cancer have been treated with cryosurgery as have patients who have had extensive prior pelvic surgery. Some patients, for a variety of reasons, choose prostate cryosurgery after a detailed and balanced discussion of all available therapies.

TECHNIQUE

The goal of prostate cryosurgery is to produce complete necrosis of the prostate gland. When achieved, this in turn produces an undetectable PSA rapidly (within 3 months) in the postoperative period (if the cancer was organ-confined). Preoperative preparation includes mechanical bowel cleansing with one or more enemas. Oral or IV antibiotics are administered preoperatively. General or spinal anesthesia can be utilized. Dorsal lithotomy position is utilized, and this can be exaggerated somewhat if pubic arch interference is encountered. Originally, when placing the larger 3-mm diameter cryoprobes, the first step was placement of the 18-gauge guide needle by hand. Currently a brachytherapy-type stereotactic grid is utilized and 17-gauge (1.7-mm diameter) "cryoneedles" are placed directly via the template grid into the prostate. Needle thermosensors are typically placed at this time as well.

Once the cryoneedles are positioned appropriately, flexible cystoscopy is used to assess the urethra, bladder neck, and bladder. Any visible cryoneedles are repositioned. Many cryosurgeons take this opportunity to place a small temporary suprapubic tube for management of the typical temporary postoperative urinary retention. Also, a urethral warming/protection device is placed at this time.

Once the preceding steps have been completed, the cryoneedles are activated, typically in an anterior to posterior sequence, with real-time monitoring by ultrasound and by temperature sensors if they are in use. As previously mentioned, there is a dramatic difference in the appearance of frozen tissue compared to normal tissue sonographically. The frozen tissue is essentially anechoic with a hyperechoic bright white boundary line between the frozen and unfrozen tissue. By closely observing these changes in multiple transverse and longitudinal planes using a bi-plane ultrasound probe, the operator can watch the freezing process unfold, and can manipulate and control the process to produce complete prostatic freezing while preserving the surrounding structures.

In addition to careful observation, a number of additional manipulations or techniques can be employed during the cryosurgical process to enhance the effectiveness and completeness of the intended prostate necrosis. Using a repeat freeze–thaw cycle is an important example of this. Both in the lab and clinically, two periods of tissue freezing separated by a period of complete or near-complete thawing will enhance the production of prostatic necrosis significantly. The attainment of very low sub-freezing temperatures appears to be important as well. While it is not possible to state a simple cut-off temperature threshold at which all prostate cells will have died, the general principle is to achieve as low a temperature as possible as quickly as possible when freezing. A nadir tissue temperature of about −40°C is thought to be adequate to kill a very high percentage of prostate cancer cells, and if this temperature is achieved twice, this enhances the effect.

Another major factor in the ability to produce complete prostatic necrosis is the placement of the cryoprobes or cryoneedles themselves. Probe placement is determined by the type of probe or needle and cryosurgical equipment which is in use. Probes (or cryoneedles) are placed in such a way that there is coverage of the entire prostate and the immediate periprostatic tissues. A discussion of specific cryoneedle placement guidelines is beyond the scope of this text, but general principles include even placement at appropriate intervals, maintenance of adequate distance from the urethra and rectum, and intelligent use of the control channels provided by the equipment in use.

The use of carefully placed tissue thermosensors as an adjunct to visual/sonographic control of freezing has be studied extensively. Especially when learning to perform prostate cryosurgery, temperature monitoring can be quite helpful, both for determining that a point within the prostate is "cold enough" as well as for determining that a point outside the prostate isn't "too cold". Needle thermosensors are placed at strategic locations in and adjacent to the prostate. One useful strategy is to place a thermosensor in a structure one wishes to preserve, such as the rectal wall or external sphincter, and then to monitor the temperature to be sure that it doesn't get too low. Another strategy is to place the thermosensor within the prostate itself to be sure that the temperature in the area monitored gets low enough. In this scenerio, one would choose an area of the prostate away from a freezing source near the periphery of the prostate, as this would be an area that would be most difficult to get to the target temperature, i.e. areas closer to the freezing source or areas more central tend to get colder quickly.

RESULTS

The ideal result of prostate cryosurgery is a patient who achieves and maintains an undetectable PSA. In addition, the ideal is to have only necrosis and fibrosis found on extensive post-cryosurgical biopsies. In our experience this result is achievable in an increasing percentage of well-selected patients treated with sound cryosurgical technique. While a detailed review of reported results of prostate cryosurgery is beyond the scope of this chapter, we will survey some literature trends, and hit some highlights from our own patient cohort. We started performing prostate cryosurgery with a five-probe liquid nitrogen system (see below) in late 1991, and as such have one of the most mature patient groups for prostate cryosurgery. This also means that our data represent a fairly long learning curve involved in the development of this procedure, which was new at the time.

Clinical local control of the primary neoplasm is achieved when there is prevention of cancer-related symptoms or morbidity caused by the local tumor. For prostate cancer, these symptoms would include problems such as obstruction, hematuria, or pain. In our experience, cryosurgery has prevented these local complications with 10-year follow-up in nearly 100% of patients with stage T1–T3 disease. Since local symptomatology generally means advanced disease, however, this clinical definition has some obvious drawbacks. Very early in the experience with percutaneous prostate cryosurgery, Cohen and Onik established systematic post-cryosurgical prostate needle biopsies as a benchmark for the assessment of local cryosurgical effect. Most investigators since then have also reported post-cryosurgical biopsies as a measure of local effectiveness. As stated above, complete necrosis of all prostate tissue is the goal of prostate cryosurgery; however, as a practical matter, some viable (benign) prostate tissue is often seen on postoperative biopsies. When viable cancer is detected on these biopsies, it is considered to represent local treatment failure. Numerous investigators have reported negative biopsy rates following cryosurgery. Three- to five-year negative rates range from 80 to 98%, as reported in the literature as well as in our own experience. At 10 years post-cryosurgery in our series of 370 patients treated primarily for T1–T3 disease, the cumulative negative biopsy rate was 65%. Despite this observation of a substantial number of positive biopsies in our earliest patients, many patients with a positive biopsy fare quite well with observation, adjuvant XRT or hormonal therapy. It is also important to note that many of our positive biopsies were from seminal vesical cores only in patients with T3 disease – the prostate being biopsy negative.

As with other therapies, serum PSA appears to be the best early surrogate endpoint of overall disease control. In the case of prostate cryosurgery, detectable postoperative PSA can be produced by benign tissue within the prostate, malignant tissue within the prostate, or malignant prostate tissue outside the prostate–metastatic disease. A variety of "biochemical control" definitions have been applied to prostate cryosurgery by investigators. The most common definition in use appears to be the RTOG criteria of three consecutive PSA rises. A newer definition which may have better applicability to prostate cryosurgery would be a nadir plus two definition. PSA nadir after prostate cryosurgery is typically achieved, unlike radiation, by 3 months after the procedure. Any increase of 2 ng/ml over the nadir value in 10 years of follow-up would be considered biochemical failure. Need for repeat cryosurgery for positive biopsy, or need for adjuvant radiation or androgen deprivation therapy would also be considered failure. Applying this definition to our cohort of 370 patients treated with cryosurgery monotherapy with a median 12.2 year follow up, the 10 year biochemical disease free survival rates were 68% for low risk patients, 74% for intermediate risk, and 36% for high risk patients. There was no statistically significant difference between the low and moderate risk group failure rates. Low risk patients had Gleason scores of <7, PSA of <10, and Stage T1 disease. High risk patients had Gleason score of >7, PSA >20, Stage T3, or more than one risk factor. The intermediate risk patients were those with Gleason score of 7, Stage T2, or PSA of 10–20 with other factors being low risk.

INTERPRETATION OF CRYOSURGERY RESULTS

When reviewing prostate cryosurgery results from the literature, it is important to bear several factors in mind. While post-cryosurgical prostate biopsies and serial longitudinal serum PSA determinations are widely used as surrogate endpoints, the interpretation of these endpoints is unsure. The issue of sampling error affects biopsy interpretation. Repeat biopsies over time will of course reduce sampling error. While an undetectable PSA is unambiguous, it is not known whether the RTOG definition of biochemical failure applies to cryosurgery in the same way that it does to radiation – the same types of analyses have not been done. This is in part why we have chosen a nadir plus two definition of biochemical failure. Anecdotally, we have numerous patients who have detectable PSAs in the 0–4 range 10 or more years out from cryosurgery who are clinically doing well with no distinct upward trend in the PSA. Many of these patients are elderly and, given their asymptomatic status, we have chosen to observe them without aggressive intervention. This strategy has worked well in our experience. With regard to the learning curve effect, post-treatment biopsy and PSA results improve with the experience of the cryosurgeon. Most of the results reported in the literature deal with the earliest series of patients treated at a given center. This of course has bearing on the results.

Cryosurgical equipment can also affect results. From 1991 to the present, there have been three main manufacturers involved in the production of cryosurgical equipment for prostate cancer. The first multichannel cryosurgical machine manufactured by Cryomedical Sciences was in use from 1991 through the late 1990s. The coolant used to drive the 3-mm cylindrical cryoprobes was supercooled liquid nitrogen. Five individual probes were available for simultaneous use. Since this was the earliest machine available, the results of treatment with it are the longest available – 10 years plus. This machine provided a powerful effective cooling source, but with a significant learning curve. In the mid 1990s, Endocare introduced a system based on the Jewell-Thompson effect of cooling with high-pressure argon gas. This machine also made use of 3-mm diameter cryoprobes, and increased the number of available probes for simultaneous use to seven. The use of the Jewell-Thompson technology allowed for more precise control of the freezing process. More recently, circa 1999, Galil Inc. (which is now Oncura) introduced a much smaller-diameter (17 gauge) cryoneedle. These smaller freezing sources could then be used with a brachytherapy-style grid/template type of arrangement for probe placement and fixation. The biggest advantage of this was ease of learning: many urologists have been trained in brachytherapy and this arrangement taps into the skill set of the urologic community gained using brachytherapy.

COMPLICATIONS

Sloughing can be described as necrosis of the prostatic urethra. This can occur in a small area, or throughout the entire surface area of the prostatic urethra. Since necrosis of prostatic stroma and glandular elements is the goal of prostate cryosurgery, this means that sloughing is basically an extension of the intended consequence of cryosurgery a few extra millimeters to a full-thickness necrosis of the relatively thin prostatic urethral mucosa. When sloughing occurs, the patient experiences frequency, dysuria, pyuria, and occasionally retentive symptomatology. When sloughing does not occur, there is generally a rapid return to normal or even improved voiding function following prostate cryosurgery. Sloughing was nearly universal prior to the use of urethral thermal protection during the procedure. In our series, sloughing occurred in 9% of patients treated with 3-mm liquid nitrogen cryoprobes and urethra protection, and is currently occurring in 1–2% of patients treated with 17 gauge cryoprobes and urethral protection. In addition to the aforementioned symptomatology, sloughing can be associated with longer-term problems such as incontinence, stricture, and calcification of the prostatic urethra. Management of sloughing is usually conservative initially with antibiotic suppression and catheter drainage as necessary. If the patient is unable to pass the necrotic tissue per urethra over time, transurethral debridement can be performed, but is best delayed at least 3 months following the initial procedure to allow for demarcation of necrotic tissue. It is clear from the literature and from our experience that sloughing is best prevented by the use of an effective urethral thermal protection device during the procedure.

Fistulization from the prostatic urethra to the rectum is one of the most severe complications reported after prostate cryosurgery. Historically, it was quite common, and was one reason why prostate cryosurgery was discontinued in the 1970s. Most contemporary series report fistula at 1% or less, with our own experience being three cases out of 1300 plus procedures. Fistulization can be a technical issue related to full-thickness freezing of the rectal muscularis and mucosa, or can be a more delayed process related to sloughing, voiding dysfunction, and bowel wall weakening from prior irradiation. Management is initially conservative with suprapubic drainage and antibiotic suppression. Some fistulas will heal spontaneously while others will need surgical intervention.

Fortunately, as with other complications associated with prostate cryosurgery, urinary incontinence has declined from historic levels. Incontinence is more likely when sloughing has occurred previously. Another risk factor would be freezing well beyond the apex of the prostate; this in turn can be monitored during the procedure using thermosensors. Patients who have had prior irradiation are at increased risk for postoperative incontinence, and many cryosurgeons are less aggressive in freezing apical tissue in this population for this reason. With current technology, our rate of permanent urinary incontinence is less than 1%. Historically, we experienced rates as high as 13% in a radiated population or if urethral thermal protection was not utilized.

Due to the nature of the freezing process, the area of frozen tissue typically extends beyond the prostatic capsule and typically involves the neurovascular bundles, especially near the apex. This in turn typically produces erectile dysfunction postoperatively. While there is certainly a delayed recovery (up to 2 years later) in up to 30% of potent patients, in general prostate cryosurgery produces permanent impotence. Several centers are currently engaged in work to develop, perfect, and test a "nerve-sparing" or "targeted" cryoablation procedure that will preserve potency. Early results are encouraging, but longer-term work is needed to see if effectiveness is equal to the standard approach.

Prostate cryosurgery inhabits a unique niche in the urologist's armamentarium in the treatment of prostate cancer. It relies neither on extirpation nor on radiation. It is minimally invasive, and provides a rapid recovery from therapy. It can produce a result similar to prostatectomy, i.e. an undetectable PSA that is durable. It has evolved greatly since its introduction in the 1960s and 1970s and to some extent is still a work in progress. It can be a welcome option, especially to patients who would not be ideally served by the other available options. Further clinical use and experience will undoubtedly further define and broaden its role moving forward.

FURTHER READING

Bahn DK, Lee F, Badalament R et al. Targeted cryoablation of the prostate: 7-year outcomes in the primary treatment of prostate cancer. Urology 2002; 60 (2 Suppl 1): 3–11.

Cohen JK, Miller RJ, Rooker GM, Shuman BA. Cryosurgical ablation of the prostate: two-year prostate specific antigen and biopsy results. Urology 1996; 47 (3): 395–401.

Donnelly JC et al. Prospective trial of cryosurgical ablation of the prostate: Five year results. Urology 2002; 60 (4): 645–9.

Flocks RH, O Donoghue PN, Milleman LA, Culp DA. Management of stage C prostate cancer urologic clinics of North America 1975; 2(1): 163–79.

Gage A. Cryosurgery. Encyclopedia of Medical Devices and Instrumentation. 1988: Vol 2: 893–908.

Gonder MJ, Soanes WA. Cryosurgical treatment of the prostate. Invest Urol 1996; 3(4): 372–8.

Han KR, Belldegrun A. Third-generation cryosurgery for primary and recurrent prostate cancer. BJU Int 2004; 93: 14–18.

Long JP, Bahn D, Lee F et al. Five-year retrospective, multi-institutional pooled analysis of cancer-related outcomes after cryosurgical ablation of the prostate. Urology 2001; 57: 518–23.

Miller RJ, Cohen JK. A closer look at cryosurgical ablation of prostate. Contemp Urol 1998; 10: 10–19.

Onik G, Porterfield B, Rubinsky B, Cohen JK. Percutaneous transperineal prostate cryosurgery using transrectal ultrasound guidance: Animal model. Urology 1991; 37 (3): 277–81.

Prepelica KL, Okeke Z, Murphy A et al. Cryosurgical ablation of prostate: high risk patient outcomes. Cancer 2005; 103 (8): 1625–30.

Sylvester JE, Blosleo JC, Grimm PD et al. Ten-year biochemical relapse-free survival after external beam radiation and brachytherapy for localized prostate cancer: the Seattle experience. Int J Radiat Oncol Biol Phys 2003; 57 (4): 944–52.

Thames H, Kuban D, Levy L et al. Comparison of alternative biochemical failure definitions based on clinical outcome in 4839 prostate cancer patients treated by external beam radiotherapy between 1986 and 1995. Int J Radiat Oncol Biol Phys 2003; 57 (4): 929–43.

Vestal CV. Critical review of the efficacy and safety of cryotherapy of the prostate. Curr Urol Rep 2005; 6 (3): 190–3.

5

Salvage cryoablation of the prostate

Sean M. Collins, Kristin Kozakowski, Aaron E. Katz

Evaluation of local recurrence after radiation therapy to the prostate • Role of hormonal therapy • Operative technique • Postoperative care • Results of salvage cryosurgery (Columbia University experience): patients • Results • Salvage radical prostatectomy • Summary

EVALUATION OF LOCAL RECURRENCE AFTER RADIATION THERAPY TO THE PROSTATE

Prostate-specific antigen (PSA) is the most sensitive measure of cancer recurrence and progression after definitive treatment of prostate cancer. After radiation therapy, PSA levels should fall slowly over 18–24 months as prostate cancer cells die from the lethal effects of radiation. The serum half-life of PSA after radiation therapy has been estimated to be 1.9 months. This is contrary to the precipitous drop in PSA levels after a successful prostatectomy, where the serum PSA half-life has been estimated to be 3.2 days. Biochemical recurrence, also known as PSA failure, is defined by the American Society of Therapeutic Radiation Oncology (ASTRO) as three consecutive rises in serum PSA with each measurement separated by 3–4 months. It is important to document three consecutive rises in PSA before diagnosing cancer recurrence, because transient rises in PSA may be seen with asymptomatic prostatitis after radiation which is know as "PSA bounce". While PSA bounce is seen more often after brachytherapy than external beam radiotherapy, it has been reported with both modalities.

PSA doubling time (PSADT) reflects tumor doubling times and the clinical aggressiveness of disease. Specifically, a PSADT less than 8 months predicts metastatic disease after radiation therapy especially if PSA begins to rise within 1 year after the completion of radiation therapy.

PSA nadir is not included in the ASTRO definition of biochemical failure. However, PSA nadirs of less than 0.5 have been shown to predict improved 5-year biochemical disease-free survival.

An ASTRO consensus panel convened in 1999 recommended that "prostate biopsy after radiation therapy is not necessary as standard follow-up care and that the absence of a rising PSA level is the most rigorous end point of total tumor eradication".

PSA failure after radiation therapy should be evaluated with a prostate biopsy however. Interpretation of a post-radiation prostate biopsy may be challenging, because radiation-induced changes in benign prostate cells may mimic prostate cancer.

A positive biopsy in a patient after radiation should prompt a metastatic work-up. CT scan of the abdomen and pelvis, bone scan, liver function test, and chest radiograph are appropriate. Radio-recurrent prostate cancer is more aggressive than primary prostate cancer, and metastases occur frequently even with relatively low PSA levels. Patients with radio-recurrent prostate cancer harbor extra-capsular disease in 40–60% of cases and nodal metastases in 14–34% of cases. Given the aggressiveness of radio recurrent prostate cancer and the poor sensitivity of CT and MRI for detecting pelvic nodal metastases from prostate cancer, laparoscopic lymphadenectomy is appropriate in this high risk population. Radiation often produces significant fibrosis which makes dissection of the pelvis and iliac vessels challenging. Therefore, post-radiation laparoscopic pelvic lymphadenectomy should be performed only by urologists with special laparoscopic expertise.

In patients who have no evidence of metastatic disease and a biopsy-proven local recurrence, cryosurgery is a treatment option.

This chapter will review salvage cryosurgery for radio-recurrent prostate cancer including the indications, techniques, outcomes, and follow-up care. Prostatectomy as an alternative treatment is also reviewed.

ROLE OF HORMONAL THERAPY

The use of neoadjuvant hormonal therapy prior to cryosurgery is still controversial. At Columbia University, hormonal therapy is routinely administered for 3 months prior to cryosurgery for the following reasons:

1. Androgen deprivation decreases the prostate gland size and thereby may improve the efficacy of cryosurgery. Reducing prostate volume increases the space between the posterior prostate capsule and the anterior rectal wall. This increased space allows for greater depth of penetration of the iceball beyond the capsule, increasing cell death in this area.
2. Despite a negative metastatic evaluation, a significant number of these high-risk patients have micrometastatic disease. Hormonal therapy may effectively treat hematogenous micrometastases, although up to 40% of distant metastases do not respond to hormonal therapy.

OPERATIVE TECHNIQUE

At Columbia University Medical Center, all cryosurgery is performed by a single surgeon. Argon and helium gases are used for freezing and thawing, respectively. A second-generation argon system is currently used. The procedure is performed under spinal anesthesia or general anesthesia according to preference of the anesthesiologist and patient. Patients receive a Fleets enema on the morning of the procedure and 500 mg of metronidazole intravenously at the start of the procedure. A 10-Fr suprapubic catheter can be placed under flexible cystoscopic guidance. The bladder is then filled with 0.9% saline and remains distended for the duration of the procedure. A urethral warming catheter is inserted before commencement of tissue freezing. The catheter is warmed to 38°C and remains in place for 2 hours after the conclusion of the procedure. Using a brachytherapy template, cryoprobes or cryoneedles are percutaneously placed into the prostate under transrectal ultrasound guidance. Thermocouple probes for temperature monitoring are placed adjacent to each of the neurovascular bundles, the apex, Denonvilliers' space, and into the external sphincter. Freezing is then initiated by activating the anterior probes, followed by the posterior probes. A double freeze–thaw technique is applied in all cases. Freezing is stopped when the outer edge of the iceball has a hyperechoic appearance and is readily visualized on transrectal ultrasound, temperature is less than $-40°C$ at each neurovascular bundle, the apical temperature is less than $-10°C$, and all prostatic tissue is frozen as visualized by ultrasound.

POSTOPERATIVE CARE

Patients are discharged home the following morning; 500 mg of ciprofloxacin is prescribed orally twice daily for 5 days. The suprapubic tube remains open and patients are instructed to clamp the tube on the fourth postoperative day. One week after the procedure, the suprapubic tube is removed. A history and physical exam is performed. Special attention is given to detect signs or symptoms of the following: perineal and scrotal swelling, ecchymosis, bladder outlet obstruction, urethral sloughing, urinary infection, and rectourethral fistula. Serum PSA is measured and digital rectal examination is performed 6 weeks after cryosurgery and every 3 months thereafter. At each follow-up, the operating surgeon evaluates morbidities. Patients are asked if they have incontinence, which is defined as patient report of lack of urinary control requiring more than 1 pad daily. Patients are also questioned about other potential complications, such as rectal pain and perineal discomfort.

RESULTS OF SALVAGE CRYOSURGERY
(COLUMBIA UNIVERSITY EXPERIENCE): PATIENTS

A retrospective analysis was performed of 195 successive patients who underwent salvage cryoablation of the prostate (SCAP) after failed radiation therapy between October 1994 and April 2005 at Columbia University Medical Center. Primary radiation therapies included 81.9% external beam radiation, 9.8% brachytherapy, and 6.7% combination external beam and brachytherapy. The mean interval between primary radiation therapy and salvage cryosurgery was 60 months (range 12–156 months). Neoadjuvant androgen-deprivation therapy was given to 82 (42.05%) patients. Adjuvant androgen deprivation was not administered unless there was evidence of disease recurrence. The mean age at cryosurgery was 69.89 years (range 50–87 years). Preoperative PSA mean and median were 6.96 ng/ml and 4.80 ng/ml (range 0–71.30 ng/ml). The median preoperative Gleason score was 7 (range of 4–10). Fifty-one patients underwent follow-up prostate biopsy.

Biochemical failure was defined by ASTRO criteria of three consecutive rises in serum PSA separated by at least 3–4 months each. Urinary retention was defined as the need for an indwelling catheter or intermittent catheterization. Patients were specifically asked about symptoms of voiding complications, rectal pain, and perineal discomfort.

RESULTS

Median follow-up was 46.5 months (range 3–128 months). During the follow-up period six (3.17%) patients died for an overall survival of 96.83%. Overall biochemical disease-free survival (bDFS) as defined by ASTRO criteria was 69.03%. The estimated 12-year cancer-specific survival and biochemical disease-free survival by

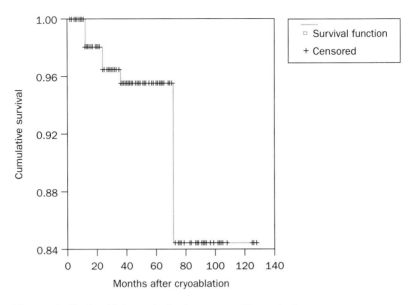

Figure 5.1   Kaplan–Meier analysis of cancer-specific survival.

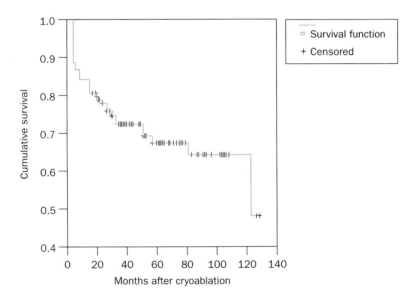

Figure 5.2   Kaplan–Meier analysis of biochemical disease-free survival by ASTRO criteria.

Kaplan–Meier analysis were greater than 80.00% and 48.21%, respectively (Figures 5.1 and 5.2). Mean and median time to failure was 17.53 and 9 months. Undetectable PSA nadir values (<0.1 ng/ml) were found in 52.88% of the population. PSA nadirs of <1.0 ng/ml and <2.0 ng/ml were found in 79.58% and 86.91%, respectively. PSA nadirs less than half of preoperative PSA were detected in 90.16% of patients.

Table 5.1 Clinical characteristics profile

	N (%)	Biochemical disease-free survival[#] (%)	PSA nadir <1.0 (%)
Gleason			
≤7	103 (52.82)	67.80	79.61
>7	92 (47.18)	70.37	76.09
PSA			
≤10 ng/ml	156 (80.00)	68.57	82.69
>10 ng/ml	39 (20.00)	73.68	53.85
XRT-SCAP interval*			
≤5 years	94 (51.37)	63.33	78.72
>5 years	89 (48.63)	81.25	76.40
Hormones			
Neoadjuvant	84 (43.08)	63.93	79.76
No hormones	111 (56.92)	75.00	74.77

Average follow-up 46.5 months (range 3–128).
*Data available for 183 patients.
[#]Biochemical failure defined as three consecutive increases in PSA separated by 3–4 months each.

Table 5.2 Morbidity by cryosurgery technology

	N	Incontinence (%)	Voiding complication (%)	Rectal pain (%)	Perineal discomfort (%)	Retention (%)
Liquid nitrogen	98	11 (11.22)	6 (6.12)	19 (19.39)	0	1 (1.02)
First-generation argon	68	2 (2.94)	3 (4.41)	1 (1.54)	3 (4.41)	2 (2.94)
Second-generation argon	29	0	0	0	0	1 (3.45)

Survival results stratified by Gleason, PSA, radiation therapy-to-salvage cryosurgery interval, and hormone status are found in Table 5.1. Significantly better bDFS was seen in those patients with an interval between XRT and salvage cryoablation of greater than 5 years and in those patients who received neoadjuvant androgen deprivation (Table 5.1).

The negative biopsy rate was 70.59% (36/51 biopsies).

Overall morbidities include 6.6% incontinence, 4.62% voiding complications, 1.54% perineal discomfort, and 2.05% retention. The most common complaint was transient rectal pain in the first 2 weeks following the procedure found in 10.26% of patients. Significantly lower rates of complications were seen in the patients treated with second-generation argon systems (Table 5.2). In these patients, the only significant complication experienced was urinary retention. There were no reports of incontinence, voiding complications, rectal pain, or perineal discomfort.

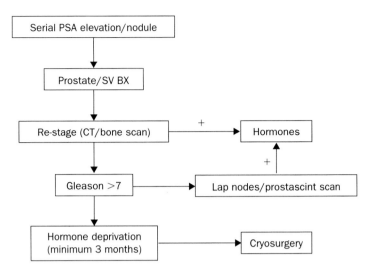

Figure 5.3   Algorithm for PSA elevations following radiation.

Table 5.3   Salvage cryosurgery: follow-up

Study	No. patients	Follow-up (months)	Biochemical recurrence	Positive prostate biopsy
Pisters 1997	150	13.5 (1.2–32.2)		25/110 (23%)
Lee 1997	43			At 3 months 3/20 (15%)
				At 1 year 7/20 (35%)
Miller 1996	33	17.1 (4.1–34.3)		9/33 (27.3%)
Present study	161	46.45 (3–128)	69.0% bRFS*	15/51 (31.0%)

*bRFS: biochemical recurrence-free survival (Kaplan–Meier curve analysis).

SALVAGE RADICAL PROSTATECTOMY

The ideal candidate for a salvage radical prostatectomy is young, healthy, and without significant medical comorbidities. He should have localized disease at the time of initial diagnosis and at the time of presentation for salvage therapy. His life expectancy should be at least 10 years. Few patients presenting for salvage treatment of radio-recurrent prostate cancer meet these criteria.

In the past, salvage prostatectomy was associated with a high incidence of rectal injury, urinary incontinence and anastomotic stricture; however, due to patient careful selection, the complication rate has decreased in recent years. Scardino et al reported morbidity associated with salvage radical prostatectomy following locally recurrent prostate cancer after radiation therapy in a series of 100 patients between 1984 and 2003. Their results showed that since 1993, the major complication rate has decreased significantly (13% vs. 33%, $P = 0.02$), including the rectal injury rate (2% vs. 15%, $P = 0.01$). Their reported 5-year continence rate was 68% requiring one daily pad or less with 23 patients undergoing artificial sphincter placement due to

Table 5.4 Salvage cryosurgery for radio-recurrent prostate cancer: comparisons of the most frequent complications reported in the literature

Study	No. patients	Incontinence (%)	Impotence (%)	Obstruction/ retention (%)	Rectal fistula (%)	Urethral strictures (%)	Pain (%)	Hydronephrosis (%)
Pisters 1997	150	60*	72***	43	1	0	NA	0
Lee 1997	46	8.7**	NA	NA	8.7	NA	NA	NA
Miller 1996	33	10.3*	NA	9	0	5.1	NA	0
Katz 2005	161	8.86*	NA	1.88	0	0	14.38	0

NA, not available.
*Incontinence = need of ≥ one pad/day.
**Incontinence = any urinary troubling.
***Preoperative potency not available.

Table 5.5 Comparison of complications of different treatment options for radio-resistant prostate cancer patients

Author	Type	No. patients	INC (%)	Obstruction (%)	Rectal injury (%)	US (%)	BR (%)
Pontes et al 1993	RP	43	30	2.3%	9	NA	60
Ahlering et al 1992	RP	11	64	NA	NA	NA	NA
Rogers et al 1995	RP	40	58	NA	15	2.5	75
Lee et al 1997	Cryo	46	9	NA	8.7	NA	53
Amling et al 1999	RP	108	23	NA	6	NA	74
Miller et al 1996	Cryo	33	9	4	0	5.1	40
Present study	Cryo	161	8.86	0	0	0	31.0

RP, radical prostatectomy; Cryo, cryosurgery; NA, not available; INC, incontinence; US, urethral sloughing; BR, biochemical recurrence.

incontinence. The anastomotic stricture rate was 30% and the 5-year potency rate was 28% following unilateral or bilateral nerve sparing RP and 45% in previously potent patients. In a study of six patients, Soloway et al reported an incontinence rate of 17% and no rectal complications.

The two largest series of salvage prostatectomies from Memorial Sloan Kettering Cancer Center & Baylor and Mayo Clinic report 10-year cancer-specific survival of 73% and 77%, respectively. Although it is difficult to make direct comparisons between studies, our estimated 12-year disease cancer-specific survival is greater than 80%. In these two salvage prostatectomy series, approximately one-third of patients were incontinent. With our current experience with modern techniques of cryosurgery, incontinence is not encountered when incontinence is defined as using greater than one pad per day.

SUMMARY

Salvage cryosurgery for radio-recurrent prostate cancer offers durable intermediate-term oncologic results. Estimated 12-year cancer-specific survival in this high-risk population is over 80%. Over two-thirds of patients remain biochemical disease-free. Complication rates have improved significantly with the introduction of improved ultrasound guidance, urethral warming devices, and second-generation argon-based systems. Rectourethral fistulae have been eliminated with modern techniques. The efficacy and side-effect profile of salvage cryosurgery compares favorably with salvage prostatectomy and is the preferred method of treating radio-recurrent, localized prostate cancer particularly in those with significant comorbidities.

FURTHER READING

Bales GT, Williams MJ, Sinner M, Thisted RA, Chodak GW. Short-term outcomes after cryosurgical ablation of the prostate in men with recurrent prostate carcinoma following radiation therapy. Urology 1995; 46: 676–80.

Baust J, Gage AA, Ma H, Zhang CM. Minimally invasive cryosurgery – technological advances. Cryobiology 1997; 34: 373–84.

Carson CC 3d, Zincke H, Utz DC et al. Radical prostatectomy after radiotherapy for prostatic cancer. J Urol 1980; 124: 237–9.

Cespedes RD, Pisters LL, von Eschenbach AC, McGuire EJ. Long-term followup of incontinence and obstruction after salvage cryosurgical ablation of the prostate: results in 143 patients. J Urol 1997; 157: 237–40.

Cox RL, Crawford ED. Complications of cryosurgical ablation of the prostate to treat localized adenocarcinoma of the prostate. Urology 1995; 45: 932–5.

Crook J, Robertson S, Esche B. Proliferative cell nuclear antigen in postradiotherapy prostate biopsies. Int J Radiat Oncol Biol Phys 1994; 30: 303–8.

Donnelly BJ, Pedersen JE, Porter AT, McPhee MS. Iridium-192 brachytherapy in the treatment of cancer of the prostate. Urol Clin North Am 1991; 18: 481–3.

Freiha FS, Bagshaw MA. Carcinoma of the prostate: results of post-irradiation biopsy. Prostate 1984; 5: 19–25.

Gill IS, Novick AC, Soble JJ et al. Laparoscopic renal cryoablation: initial clinical series. Urology 1998; 52: 543–51.

Goldstone LM, Scardino PT. Salvage radical prostatectomy for radiorecurrent adenocarcinoma of the prostate. J Urol 1990; 143: 220A.

Harper DM, Cobb JL. Cervical mucosal block effectively reduces the pain and cramping from cryosurgery. J Fam Pract 1998; 47: 285–9.

Kabalin JN, Hodge KK, McNeal JE et al. Identification of residual cancer in the prostate following radiation therapy: role of transrectal ultrasound guided biopsy and prostate specific antigen. J Urol 1989; 142: 326–31.

Kiesling VJ, McAninch JW, Goebel JL, Agee RE. External beam radiotherapy for adenocarcinoma of the prostate: a clinical followup. J Urol 1980; 124: 851–4.

Lee F, Bahn DK, McHugh TA et al. Cryosurgery of prostate cancer. Use of adjuvant hormonal therapy and temperature monitoring – A one year follow-up. Anticancer Res 1997; 17: 1511–15.

Lee F, Torp-Pedersen S, Meiselman L et al. Transrectal ultrasound in the diagnosis and staging of local disease after I125 seed implantation for prostate cancer. Int J Radiat Oncol Biol Phys 1988; 15: 1453–9.

Link P, Freiha FS. Radical prostatectomy after definitive radiation therapy for prostate cancer. Urology 1991; 37: 189–92.

Malawer MM, Bickels J, Meller I et al. Cryosurgery in the treatment of giant cell tumor. A long-term followup study. Clin Orthop 1999; 359: 176–88.

Maroon JC, Onik G, Quigley MR et al. Cryosurgery re-visited for the removal and destruction of brain, spinal and orbital tumours. Neurol Res 1992; 14: 294–302.

Mettlin CJ, Murphy G. The National Cancer Data Base report on prostate cancer. Cancer 1994; 74: 1640–8.

Miller RJ Jr, Cohen JK, Shuman B, Merlotti LA. Percutaneous, transperineal cryosurgery of the prostate as salvage therapy for post radiation recurrence of adenocarcinoma. Cancer 1996; 77: 1510–14.

Onik GM, Cohen JK, Reyes GD et al. Transrectal ultrasound-guided percutaneous radical cryosurgical ablation of the prostate. Cancer 1993; 72: 1291–9.

Patel BG, Parsons CL, Bidair M, Schmidt JD. Cryoablation for carcinoma of the prostate. J Surg Oncol 1996; 63: 256–64.

Pisters LL, von Eschenbach AC, Scott SM et al. The efficacy and complications of salvage cryotherapy of the prostate. J Urol 1997; 157: 921–5.

Prestidge BR, Kaplan I, Cox RS, Bagshaw MA. Predictors of survival after a positive post-irradiation prostate biopsy. Int J Radiat Oncol Biol Phys 1994; 28: 17–22.

Rogers E, Ohori M, Kassabian VS et al. Salvage radical prostatectomy: outcome measured by serum prostate specific antigen levels. J Urol 1995; 153: 104–10.

Schellhammer PF, el-Mahdi AM, Higgins EM et al. Prostate biopsy after definitive treatment by interstitial 125-iodine implant or external beam radiation therapy. J Urol 1987; 137: 897–901.

Shinohara K, Connolly JA, Presti JC Jr, Carroll PR. Cryosurgical treatment of localized prostate cancer (stages T1 to T4): preliminary results. J Urol 1996; 156: 115–20.

Zegel HG, Holland GA, Jennings SB et al. Intraoperative ultrasonographically guided cryoablation of renal masses: initial experience. J Ultrasound Med 1998; 17: 571–6.

6

Focal cryoablation of the prostate: patient-specific modifications of ultrasound-guided prostatic cryoablation

Daniel B. Rukstalis

Introduction • **Multifocal cancer and tumor volume** • **Patient-specific modifications of focal cryoablation** • **Imaging of prostate cryoablation** • **Technique of focal prostate cryoablation** • **Conclusions**

INTRODUCTION

The percutaneous transperineal placement of small metal probes into the prostate under transrectal ultrasound guidance represents the most flexible therapeutic method for the destruction of prostatic cancer. Since the initial description of an animal model for ultrasound-guided cryoablation in 1991 this technique was designed to eradicate clinically localized prostate cancer through the destruction of the entire prostate.[1] Treatment approaches, which now include computer-guided treatment-planning software, focused on the placement of 5–8 cryoprobes in an array that would result in the entire prostate gland becoming engulfed in lethal ice. This lethal ice, with a temperature below −20 to −40°C, would injure and ultimately ablate prostatic tissue through a combination of direct cellular injury and vascular occlusion. The challenge of such an approach is to limit the destructive effects of the treatment to the prostate while sparing tissue such as the urethra, rectum, and neurovascular bundles. As always, the clinical challenge is to balance treatment efficacy against associated treatment-related toxicity.

Clinical investigators have attempted to address this challenge in a manner similar to the approach taken with the radical prostatectomy and radiation therapy. Modifications in the surgical technique of the radical prostatectomy have served to spare the periprostatic tissue, when appropriate, with nerve-sparing, bladder neck-sparing and even urethral-sparing approaches. Radiation oncologists have developed ever more accurate imaging and delivery systems designed to escalate the dose of radiation to the prostate while limiting the dose to the surrounding tissue: in effect, performing a bladder-, urethra-, and rectal-sparing therapy.

Clinicians, investigators, and manufacturers are also engaged in a similar developmental process with prostatic cryoablation. The ability of ultrasound to provide real-time information about treatment planning and performance facilitates the process of tissue sparing with this technique. This chapter is designed to address the rationale for the destruction of the entire prostate followed by a scientific foundation for the development of more individualized treatment approaches that spare some tissue in order to better balance treatment efficacy and toxicity.

MULTIFOCAL CANCER AND TUMOR VOLUME

The pathologic examination of a radical prostatectomy specimen often demonstrates multiple distinct lesions within the prostate. The incidence of multifocal cancer varies between 50 and 80% and this finding represents the single most important reason for a total gland treatment for clinically localized prostate cancer.[2,3] Furthermore, prostatic adenocarcinoma likely results from a field defect within the luminal epithelium, which also supports the therapeutic strategy of total gland ablation with surgical extirpation or *in situ* destruction. However, since any treatment designed to destroy the entire prostate gland also injures adjacent tissues such as the neurovascular bundles, bladder neck, and rectum these treatments are associated with an unavoidable rate of adverse events. Therefore, ongoing efforts designed to balance the desire to eradicate the localized cancer with a reduction in treatment-related side effects must consider methods for avoiding injury to the periprostatic tissue. This balance can only be achieved if the volume of prostate cancer present at the time of diagnosis is small enough and adequately localized to facilitate a reduction in the degree of tissue destruction needed to eradicate it. Current clinical efforts with early detection programs using serum prostate specific antigen and improved prostate biopsy templates appear to result in the identification of smaller-volume prostate cancers. Therefore, the flexibility of ultrasound-guided percutaneous prostate cryoablation may be suited for specific *in situ* tissue-sparing approaches.

Stamey and co-workers started the scientific effort to determine prostate cancer volume and its relationship to treatment outcomes with the evaluation of 139 consecutive normal prostate glands removed as part of a radical cystoprostatectomy.[3] These investigators determined that 55 of the 139 men (40%) harbored prostate cancer, which was coincident with the rate of prostate cancer found in men on autopsy. Furthermore, the total cancer volume, provided by a sum of the volume of each individual focus, ranged between 0.5 and 6.1 ml with 80% of the tumors less than $0.5\,cm^3$ in volume. The authors concluded that prostate cancers with a total volume of $0.5\,cm^3$ or less are not likely to reach a clinically significant volume within an individual man's lifetime. Therefore, only cancers with a volume larger than 0.5 ml should be targeted for therapy.

The concept that a cancer volume of less than $0.5\,cm^3$ represents the tipping point between intervention and observation has become an accepted position within the urologic community. This concept is often applied in the literature to calculate the need for therapy in an individual patient. However, neither transrectal ultrasound nor sextant prostate biopsy can accurately predict cancer volume limiting the value of using cancer volume estimates in determining optimum treatment.[4,5] This clinical conundrum has become more challenging as the overall cancer volume within the prostates of men, at the time of diagnosis, with prostate cancer has progressively decreased from approximately $4–5\,cm^3$ to $1–2\,cm^3$ over the past decade. Furthermore, the decline in the volume of the index cancer has been associated with a reduction in the number and volume of the ancillary cancers. This appears to be the impact of PSA-based early detection programs and a paradigm shift towards an increased number of biopsy cores obtained at the time of initial prostate biopsy.

Many clinical investigators have examined the pathologic appearance of prostate cancer in radical prostatectomy specimens obtained in the modern PSA era.

These studies have continued to demonstrate the multifocality of prostate cancer. However, it appears that an increasing number of men present with unifocal cancer or total cancer volumes below $0.5\,cm^3$. In particular, Ward and co-workers examined the prostate glands from men treated with a cystoprostatectomy for bladder cancer in the setting of a serum PSA between 0 and $2\,ng/ml$.[6] A total of 40% of men harbored a clinically insignificant cancer if the definition of significant cancer included any factor such as a cancer volume greater than $0.5\,cm^3$, Gleason 4 or 5 architecture, positive margins, non-diploid nuclear content, and multifocality greater than three sites. This finding appears to be consistent with other investigations that examine the results of extended prostate needle biopsy templates. Epstein and others evaluated a total of 103 radical prostatectomy specimens taken from men who were predicted to have small-volume or clinically insignificant cancer preoperatively based on a saturation biopsy approach. The median total cancer volume at radical prostatectomy in this group was $0.14\,cm^3$. Although the authors concluded that the saturation biopsy approach was adequate for predicting clinically significant cancer, the overall cancer volume was low and 11% of men still fit the definition of insignificant cancer.[7] Importantly, these patients still elected to receive curative therapy with a radical prostatectomy and could be candidates for alternative treatment approaches beyond watchful waiting.

Transrectal ultrasound-guided prostate biopsy protocols have improved the ability to detect and localize prostate cancer. A template for random systematic sextant biopsies was initially developed in 1989 and resulted in a cancer detection rate as high as 66% in men with abnormal findings on a digital rectal examination.[8–10] Since that time many articles have been published demonstrating the improved detection rate and prognostic ability of extended core biopsy approaches. Presti and co-workers have evaluated 8-, 10-, and 12-core approaches with a focus on the lateral and anterior horn of the peripheral zone.[11–13] In general, the diagnostic yield for prostate cancer is increased when more cores are obtained from the peripheral zone. Furthermore, information from patient series comparing prostate needle biopsy results to the histopathologic findings on radical prostatectomy has suggested that algorithms which include the number of positive cores and the length of cancer on an involved biopsy specimen may predict the presence of clinically significant cancer.[7] Although such a predictive ability would be beneficial for patients considering focal ablative therapies there are at least two series with a total of 519 men that found the correlation between biopsy results and the presence of significant cancer to be weak.[14,15] Clinical investigators who have pushed the number of biopsy core specimens as high as 20–100 cores using specialized transperineal and transrectal biopsy protocols further demonstrate this mathematical reality. Ficarra and associates have demonstrated a cancer detection rate of 40–43% using a 10–14-core transperineal prostate biopsy procedure.[16] Pinkstaff and others demonstrated that the transperineal biopsy technique identifies

Table 6.1 Results of prostate needle biopsy patient series

Author	Date	No. men	No. cores	No. pos	Unilateral/unifocal
Epstein	2005	56	44 (24–54)	3 (1–21)	73% ($<0.5\,cm^3$)
Chan	2001	297	3–18	2.6 (1–12)	29% unifocal
Noguchi	2001	222	6.4 (6–13)	2.1 (1–7)	73%/35.1%
Terris	1992	124	6	NA	21.7% unifocal

Table 6.2   Results of radical prostatectomy series

Author	Date	No.	Stage	Cancer volume	Significant (%)	Insignificant (%)
Chan	2001	297	NA	1.6 cm³	75.6	24.4
Noguchi	2001	222	T1c	1.86 cm³	90	10
Carter	1997	168	T1c	NA		69 (PSA<4)
						33 (PSA<5)
Stamey	1998	791	T1a–T2c	2.4 cm³ (T1c)		
				1.8 cm³ (T2a)		
				4.1 cm³ (T2b)		
				5.5 cm³ (T2c)		

a higher percentage of the transition zone cancers than does the more traditional transrectal approach.[17] Additionally, a prospective comparison of the transperineal versus the transrectal approach demonstrated a 15–20% diagnostic improvement of the transperineal approach over a transrectal biopsy technique.[18] Since the volume of prostate cancer at the time of diagnosis appears to be related to the number of biopsy cores performed, it is likely that the increased diagnostic yield of the transperineal technique will result in an increased diagnosis of unilateral, unifocal, and small-volume cancers. Crawford and co-workers who have developed a computer model for assessing the diagnostic accuracy of transperineal biopsy approaches with either a 5 mm or 10 mm distance between the biopsy sites further demonstrate this phenomenon. They found that the transperineal biopsy technique with 5 mm spacing between each biopsy site resulted in a 66% diagnostic rate with as many as 108 cores performed. Importantly, the authors found that this approach was able to detect, and potentially predict, three-quarters of the unilateral cancers.[19] This suggests that men with low-volume unilateral prostate cancer may be identified more accurately and therefore qualify for focal prostatic ablation rather than whole-gland therapy.

PATIENT-SPECIFIC MODIFICATIONS OF FOCAL CRYOABLATION

The technique of transperineal cryoablation of the prostate for prostatic adenocarcinoma was significantly advanced in 1988 when the ultrasound appearance of the therapeutic iceball was first described.[20] The hyperechoic leading edge of the ice within the prostate was easily visualized. This provided the opportunity to use transrectal ultrasound to guide the accurate placement of needles into the prostate and to control the extension of the ice throughout the prostate and periprostatic tissues. Prostate cryoablation has been developed as a whole-gland treatment much like other established modalities such as external-beam radiation therapy and brachytherapy.[21] Clinical investigators have demonstrated the successful ablation of the entire prostate with acceptable morbidity coupled with a low incidence of residual cancer on follow-up biopsies.[22–24]

The advent of argon gas-based cryoablation equipment has further reduced the treatment-related toxicities while facilitating the accurate placement of cryoprobes.[25,26] Furthermore, computer-guided treatment planning software has resulted in a more detailed treatment plan with the ability to specifically target regions of the prostate in an effort to maintain treatment efficacy and reduce adverse events.[27] Prospective quality-of-life trials have heightened the intensity with which adverse events are viewed for a population of men with smaller and more localized prostatic cancers.[28–30] In particular, sexually active men are highly motivated to maintain spontaneous erectile function and appear to favor treatment options that maximize this outcome. Together with the increased identification of unilateral prostate cancer, the desire on the part of patients and their treating physicians to minimize treatment-related erectile dysfunction and incontinence has stimulated modifications of the whole-gland cryoablation technique. These modifications have been called focal ablation, individualized or patient specific, as well as the male lumpectomy.[31,32]

The concept of focal ablation describes the creation of a patient-specific individualized treatment plan, which results in the destruction of the known cancer while avoiding injury to otherwise healthy anatomic structures. Ultrasound-guided transperineal prostate cryoablation is the only treatment option with the inherent technical flexibility for such individualized treatment planning. Onik and co-workers published in 2002 a series of nine men treated with focal prostatic ablation described as the destruction of the side ipsilateral to the positive biopsy.[31] None of the men developed incontinence while seven of nine maintained normal erotic erectile function. Importantly, six of six men had negative follow-up prostate biopsies and the group exhibited stable PSA levels with a mean of 36 months of clinical monitoring.

The ability to target specific regions of the prostate also implies the capacity to protect other vital regions of intraprostatic and periprostatic tissue. The modern technique of prostate cryoablation has long incorporated urethral warming to avoid urethral injury.[33] Although this approach may risk sparing cancer that is located adjacent to the urethral wall the clinical imperative to balance efficacy and toxicity has supported this strategy.[2,34] Similarly, urethral-sparing and nerve-sparing modifications have been made to the standard radical prostatectomy and brachytherapy in the name of minimizing adverse events. It may also be possible to perform nerve-sparing cryoablation by the intentional placement of a warming probe in the region of the neurovascular bundle. Janzen and co-investigators evaluated active warming of the neurovascular bundles in a canine model which demonstrated the ability to ablate prostatic tissue while minimizing injury to the bundles.[35] Importantly, four of seven prostatic lobes adjacent to the warmed bundles revealed partially intact parenchyma. Therefore, intentional nerve-sparing prostate cryoablation is likely to represent another version of the individualized approach to treating prostate cancer, which will leave some portion of the prostatic parenchyma untreated.

Focal cryoablation is first and foremost a statistical balancing act between cancer ablation and the risk of injury to adjacent structures. Rukstalis and co-investigators attempted to use information from the evaluation of 112 consecutive sagittally sectioned whole-mounted radical prostatectomy specimens to predict the likelihood of cancer ablation during a focal prostatic ablation procedure.[2] Prostate cancer was multifocal in 79.5% of cases with a median index cancer volume of $1.6\,cm^3$ and a median ancillary cancer volume of $0.3\,cm^3$. When the prostate was conceptually divided into 12 zones, described as bilateral anterior and posterior apex, mid and base, the likelihood of cancer eradication could be estimated relative to the number of zones ablated. In particular, if nine zones were ablated the likelihood of eradicating all significant cancer was 80–90%. This mathematical prediction has been recapitulated in our clinical experience with individualized prostate cryoablation. The positive biopsy rate following focal cryoablation in an unpublished series of 102 men has been 21%. In each instance, the residual cancer has been <5% of one core and located on the side contralateral to the index cancer.

IMAGING OF PROSTATE CRYOABLATION

Successful focal ablation of a specific cancer site within the prostate will remain a statistical exercise until improvements in imaging take place that allow a more detailed localization of an individual cancer. Several imaging modalities appear to be likely candidates for technological improvements. These include magnetic resonance imaging (MRI), magnetic resonance spectroscopy (MRS), positron emission tomography (PET), endorectal power Doppler ultrasound, and contrast-enhanced Doppler ultrasound.[36]

Contrast-enhanced MRI has been found to accurately represent the extent of necrosis within the ablation zone in the prostate following cryoablation.[37] In one study, men received a minimally invasive ablation for prostate cancer followed by a gadolinium-enhanced MRI and a subsequent radical prostatectomy for histologic comparison. The MRI images correlated well with the visual size and location of the ablation zone, suggesting that this modality may provide information regarding efficacy of an ablation procedure.[37] The combination of MRI and MRS has demonstrated the ability to identify prostate cancer in animal models.[38,39] Clinical investigators have found that the combination also appears to improve the localization of cancer within the prostate of men.[40] In particular, dynamic contrast-enhanced MRI imaging was found to provide excellent demarcation of the cancer borders in 90% of men in one study.[41] It appears that MRI techniques may be useful in the future for directing prostate core biopsies, determining the application of focal ablation and postoperative assessment of the ablation zone.

Transrectal ultrasound is the most likely candidate for technologic innovation since all current ablative procedures have incorporated ultrasound into the technique. Gray-scale ultrasound is an insensitive tool for localizing individual prostate cancers since the majority of lesions are isoechoic to the normal prostatic parenchyma. Doppler and power Doppler ultrasounds have the ability to identify hypervascular regions within the prostate, which may harbor cancer. In one series of 85 men contrast-enhanced color Doppler ultrasound had a 93% sensitivity and an 87% specificity for cancer on biopsy.[42] Contrast-enhanced color Doppler ultrasound demonstrated a sensitivity of 50.8% and a specificity of 95.2% in another series of 18 patients, 15 with biopsy-proven prostate cancer.[43] These patient series suggest that Doppler ultrasound and contrast-enhanced color Doppler ultrasound can improve the detection rate of prostate cancer while also providing improved localization of specific cancers for focal ablation. Although all current imaging modalities are unable to identify microscopic foci of cancer it is likely that these foci are not clinically significant at the time of treatment of the larger index cancer. Since prostate cryoablation is easily repeated without additional patient-related toxicity it appears reasonable to target each focus of cancer individually.

TECHNIQUE OF FOCAL PROSTATE CRYOABLATION

The technical focus of a focal or individualized prostate cryoablation is to reliably destroy some portion of the prostate while sparing adjacent parenchyma. In particular, the procedure is performed under transrectal ultrasound guidance in a fashion similar to the total or standard prostate cryoablation procedure except that the cryo-probes are placed in the area of the cancer identified on the preoperative prostate biopsy. Furthermore, the cryoprobes are positioned in such a fashion as to minimize injury to the circumference of the urethra, the contralateral neurovascular, and/or the external sphincter.

Onik and co-workers published an initial report in 2002 which included a description of their operative approach.[31] The technique was individualized with probe placement tailored to the patient based on prostatic anatomy, tumor location, clinical grade, and stage. The neurovascular bundle was intentionally destroyed on the side ipsilateral to the known cancer. Cryoprobes were placed 1.0 cm apart and within 5 mm of the prostatic capsule on the side of the tumor. It appeared that these authors most often destroyed at least six zones, or the entire side ipsilateral to the cancer using an argon gas-based system.

There are currently no other published reports of the surgical technique for focal prostatic cryoablation. Our own experience with the technique is similar to that published by Onik and employs a transrectal ultrasound-guided approach for the placement of cryoprobes through a brachytherapy-type grid system in such a fashion as to destroy the majority of prostate tissue while avoiding injury to the contralateral neurovascular bundle and external sphincter. In an unpublished experience the procedure has been performed as an outpatient in more than 100 men with a median urethral catheter dwell time of 3 days. There have been no major complications in our patient series.

Importantly, the optimal candidates for a focal or individualized cryoablation remain uncertain. There is an inherent risk for every man who elects to receive a parenchymal-sparing procedure in an effort to minimize treatment-related side effects. The majority of men with prostate cancer harbor a multifocal cancer within the prostate irrespective of the information provided by preoperative imaging studies or the prostate biopsy. However, sizable minorities, often as many as 35%, of men are found to have a small-volume and unifocal cancer on radical prostatectomy. These represent the men who could receive a focal ablation with a reasonable expectation of complete eradication of their cancer. A large longitudinal study of serum PSA levels in a population of men receiving regular prostatic cancer early detection examinations found that for men with a PSA less than 4.0 ng/ml the majority (69%) were less than 0.5 cm^3. In the men with a serum PSA below 5.0 ng/ml the percentile of small cancers was 33%.[44] It is these men who would benefit most from a minimally invasive treatment for their cancers. Additionally, it appears that the incidence of small-volume and unifocal cancers is highest in the group of men with only 1–2 out of 8–13 biopsy cores involved with cancer. Therefore, current evidence would identify the men with a small cancer on biopsy, without any Gleason 4 or 5 patterns and a PSA less than 5.0 ng/ml, as the best candidates for focal therapy.

CONCLUSIONS

Ultrasound-guided transperineal prostatic cryoablation is a highly flexible and efficacious treatment option for men with clinically localized prostate adenocarcinoma. Technological improvements in the cryoablation equipment coupled with an apparent trend towards the diagnosis of smaller-volume and unifocal cancers have provided the impetus for the development of individualized treatment plans. The focal ablation of the known cancer can now be accomplished with a reduced risk of injury to adjacent anatomic structures such as the urethra, intrinsic urethral sphincter, and the neurovascular bundles. This concept is highly attractive to men with prostate cancer who desire therapy but have been educated about the protracted natural history of most prostate cancers. The ongoing evolution towards a better transrectal or transperineal biopsy technique has increased the likelihood that a prostate cancer will be detected at a smaller volume making focal ablation more attractive to these patients.

However, optimism is not a sufficient reason to pursue a new treatment modality. Important questions about efficacy and cost remain unanswered. Several single-institution patient series are likely to be published in the near future and may provide some of these answers. Incomplete destruction of the prostate is likely to obviate the clinical usefulness of the postoperative serum PSA value for clinical follow-up much in the same manner as with radiation therapeutic options. Therefore, a follow-up prostate biopsy is important for all men treated with the focal approach. Additionally, current imaging techniques are unable to specifically localize the individual index cancer in a manner that will insure complete ablation. Therefore, focal ablation must be individualized with a consideration of zones of destruction until better imaging is available. Many men with prostate cancer will find the focal ablative approach attractive even if it means that several procedures are required over the time frame of their treatment for prostate cancer.

REFERENCES

1. Onik G, Porterfield B, Rubinsky B, Cohen J. Percutaneous transperineal prostate cryosurgery using transrectal ultrasound guidance: animal model. Urology 1991; 37: 277–81.
2. Rukstalis DB, Goldknopf JL, Crowley EM, Garcia FU. Prostate cryoablation: a scientific rationale for future modifications. Urology 2002; 60: 19–25.
3. Stamey TA, Freiha FS, McNeal JE et al. Localized prostate cancer. Relationship of tumor volume to clinical significance for treatment of prostate cancer. Cancer 1993; 71: 933–8.
4. Terris MK, McNeal JE, Stamey TA. Estimation of prostate cancer volume by transrectal ultrasound imaging. J Urol 1992; 147: 855–7.
5. Terris MK, Haney DJ, Johnstone IM et al. Prediction of prostate cancer volume using prostate-specific antigen levels, transrectal ultrasound, and systematic sextant biopsies. Urology 1995; 45: 75–80.
6. Ward JF, Bartsch G, Sebo TJ et al. Pathologic characterization of prostate cancers with a very low serum prostate specific antigen (0–2 ng/mL) incidental to cystoprostatectomy: is PSA a useful indicator of clinical significance? Urol Oncol 2004; 22: 40–7.
7. Epstein JI, Sanderson H, Carter HB, Scharfstein DO. Utility of saturation biopsy to predict insignificant cancer at radical prostatectomy. Urology 2005; 66: 356–60.
8. Hodge KK, McNeal JE, Terris MK, Stamey TA. Random systematic versus directed ultrasound guided transrectal core biopsies of the prostate. J Urol 1989; 142: 71–4; discussion 74–5.
9. Hodge KK, McNeal JE, Stamey TA. Ultrasound guided transrectal core biopsies of the palpably abnormal prostate. J Urol 1989; 142: 66–70.
10. Epstein JI, Lecksell K, Carter HB. Prostate cancer sampled on sextant needle biopsy: significance of cancer on multiple cores from different areas of the prostate. Urology 1999; 54: 291–4.
11. Meng MV, Franks JH, Presti JC Jr, Shinohara K. The utility of apical anterior horn biopsies in prostate cancer detection. Urol Oncol 2003; 21: 361–5.
12. Presti JC Jr. Prostate biopsy: how many cores are enough? Urol Oncol 2003; 21: 135–40.

13. Chon CH, Lai FC, McNeal JE, Presti JC Jr. Use of extended systematic sampling in patients with a prior negative prostate needle biopsy. J Urol 2002; 167: 2457–60.
14. Noguchi M, Stamey TA, McNeal JE, Yemoto CM. Relationship between systematic biopsies and histological features of 222 radical prostatectomy specimens: lack of prediction of tumor significance for men with nonpalpable prostate cancer. J Urol 2001; 166: 104–9; discussion 109–10.
15. Chan TY, Chan DY, Stutzman KL, Epstein JI. Does increased needle biopsy sampling of the prostate detect a higher number of potentially insignificant tumors? J Urol 2001; 166: 2181–4.
16. Ficarra V, Novella G, Novara G et al. The potential impact of prostate volume in the planning of optimal number of cores in the systematic transperineal prostate biopsy. Eur Urol 2005; 48: 932–7.
17. Pinkstaff DM, Igel TC, Petrou SP et al. Systematic transperineal ultrasound-guided template biopsy of the prostate: three-year experience. Urology 2005; 65: 735–9.
18. Emiliozzi P, Corsetti A, Tassi B et al. Best approach for prostate cancer detection: a prospective study on transperineal versus transrectal six-core prostate biopsy. Urology 2003; 61: 961–6.
19. Crawford ED, Wilson SS, Torkko KC et al. Clinical staging of prostate cancer: a computer-simulated study of transperineal prostate biopsy. BJU Int 2005; 96: 999–1004.
20. Onik G, Cobb C, Cohen J et al. US characteristics of frozen prostate. Radiology 1988; 168: 629–31.
21. Lee F, Bahn DK, McHugh TA et al. US-guided percutaneous cryoablation of prostate cancer. Radiology 1994; 192: 769–76.
22. Donnelly BJ, Saliken J, McDougall L, Temple WJ. Pilot study to determine safety and short-term outcome of percutaneous cryoablation in the treatment of localized prostate cancer (stages T1C-T3C NO MO). Can J Urol 1996; 3: 261–7.
23. Long JP, Bahn D, Lee F et al. Five-year retrospective, multi-institutional pooled analysis of cancer-related outcomes after cryosurgical ablation of the prostate. Urology 2001; 57: 518–23.
24. Bahn DK, Lee F, Badalament R et al. Targeted cryoablation of the prostate: 7-year outcomes in the primary treatment of prostate cancer. Urology 2003; 60: 3–11.
25. Zisman A, Pantuck AJ, Cohen JK, Belldegrun AS. Prostate cryoablation using direct transperineal placement of ultrathin probes through a 17-gauge brachytherapy template-technique and preliminary results. Urology 2001; 58: 988–93.
26. Ellis DS. Cryosurgery as primary treatment for localized prostate cancer: a community hospital experience. Urology 2002; 60: 34–9.
27. Wojtowicz A, Selman S, Jankun J. Computer simulation of prostate cryoablation – fast and accurate approximation of the exact solution. Comput Aided Surg 2003; 8: 91–7.
28. Anastasiadis AG, Sachdev R, Salomon L et al. Comparison of health-related quality of life and prostate-associated symptoms after primary and salvage cryotherapy for prostate cancer. J Cancer Res Clin Oncol 2003; 129: 676–82.
29. Robinson JW, Saliken JC, Donnelly BJ et al. Quality-of-life outcomes for men treated with cryosurgery for localized prostate carcinoma. Cancer 1999; 86: 1793–801.
30. Robinson JW, Donnelly BJ, Saliken JC et al. Quality of life and sexuality of men with prostate cancer 3 years after cryosurgery. Urology 2002; 60: 12–18.
31. Onik G, Narayan P, Vaughan D et al. Focal "nerve-sparing" cryosurgery for treatment of primary prostate cancer: a new approach to preserving potency. Urology 2002; 60: 109–14.
32. Onik G. The male lumpectomy: rationale for a cancer targeted approach for prostate cryoablation. A review. Technol Cancer Res Treat 2004; 3: 365–70.
33. Cohen JK, Miller RJ, Shuman BA. Urethral warming catheter for use during cryoablation of the prostate. Urology 1995; 45: 861–4.
34. Leibovich BC, Blute ML, Bostwick DG et al. Proximity of prostate cancer to the urethra: implications for minimally invasive ablative therapies. Urology 2000; 56: 726–9.

35. Janzen NK, Han KR, Perry KT et al. Feasibility of nerve-sparing prostate cryosurgery: applications and limitations in a canine model. J Endourol 2005; 19: 520–5.
36. Hersh MR, Knapp EL, Choi J. Newer imaging modalities to assess tumor in the prostate. Cancer Control 2004; 11: 353–7.
37. Larson BT, Collins JM, Huidobro C et al. Gadolinium-enhanced MRI in the evaluation of minimally invasive treatments of the prostate: correlation with histopathologic findings. Urology 2003; 62: 900–4.
38. Fricke ST, Rodriguez O, Vanmeter J et al. In vivo magnetic resonance volumetric and spectroscopic analysis of mouse prostate cancer models. Prostate 2006; 66: 708–17.
39. Fan X, Medved M, Foxley S et al. Multi-slice DCE-MRI data using P760 distinguishes between metastatic and non-metastatic rodent prostate tumors. MAGMA 2006; 19: 15–21.
40. Huzjan R, Sala E, Hricak H. Magnetic resonance imaging and magnetic resonance spectroscopic imaging of prostate cancer. Nat Clin Pract Urol 2005; 2: 434–42.
41. Kim CK, Park BK, Kim B. Localization of prostate cancer using 3T MRI: comparison of T2-weighted and dynamic contrast-enhanced imaging. J Comput Assist Tomogr 2006; 30: 7–11.
42. Roy C, Buy X, Lang H et al. Contrast enhanced color Doppler endorectal sonography of prostate: efficiency for detecting peripheral zone tumors and role for biopsy procedure. J Urol 2003; 170: 69–72.
43. Strohmeyer D, Frauscher F, Klauser A et al. Contrast-enhanced transrectal color doppler ultrasonography (TRCDUS) for assessment of angiogenesis in prostate cancer. Anticancer Res 2001; 21: 2907–13.
44. Carter HB, Epstein JI, Chan DW et al. Recommended prostate-specific antigen testing intervals for the detection of curable prostate cancer. JAMA 1997; 277: 1456–60.

7

Quality of life following prostate cryoablation

Jennifer Simmons

Any discussion of treatment modalities for prostate cancer includes a dissertation on what the patient might expect to experience after treatment. Most patients diagnosed with prostate cancer have localized disease and are candidates for several different treatments. In addition, prostate cancer has a long natural history, and is being diagnosed in earlier stages, and so most patients are expected to live with the effects of their treatment for many years.

The side effects of various treatments for prostate cancer have been studied for decades, but attention is increasingly shifting to assessing the impact of these side effects on quality of life. These studies have illustrated that for most patients, actively combating their disease leads to an improved sense of well-being, and certain side effects lower the quality of life more than others.

Tools are emerging which reliably capture quality-of-life data. Surveys developed to assess health-related quality of life have been modified to capture information pertinent to prostate cancer treatment such as urinary and bowel symptoms, and erectile dysfunction.

It is well established that data gathered by physician interview of a patient tend to underestimate side effects.[1] Ideally data should be collected via patient-completed validated questionnaires. There are several questionnaires available for use in prostate cancer patients. Surveys can be broken down into domains. Generic quality-of-life domains assess general health areas. Disease-specific domains study side effects associated with the disease or procedure of study. The domains relevant to prostate cancer and its treatment include bladder continence, erectile function, bladder irritation, bowel function, worry about cancer control, and hot flashes.[2]

One such survey is the Functional Assessment of Cancer Treatment-Prostate (FACT-P).[3,4] It is a survey composed of the 28 question FACT tool developed for general cancer patients with 12 items added to evaluate prostate cancer-specific domains. The generic domains include Physical, Social/Family, Emotional Well-Being, Functional Well-Being, and Relationship with Doctor. Prostate-specific domains include Appetite/Weight, Pain, Bladder Function, Bowel Function, and Sexual Function.

Robinson et al used the FACT-P to study 69 men undergoing prostate cryotherapy as primary treatment of localized prostate cancer in Canada. Participants were asked to complete the survey pretreatment and at 6 weeks, 3 months, 6 months, and 12 months after therapy. At 6 weeks, quality-of-life total score was significantly lower than pretreatment. Steady recovery was noted subsequently and at the final survey, total scores were not different from baseline. Within individual domains, physical, social, and functional well-being scores followed a similar trend of decrease at 6 weeks followed by normalization by 12 months. The social well-being domain score did not return to baseline at 12 months, but the difference did not reach statistical significance, defined as $P < 0.01$. Emotional well-being showed a different trend altogether, with the lowest score at the pretreatment survey, with significantly higher scores at 6 weeks, which persisted through to 12 months. The prostate-specific domain showed a similar pattern of nadir at 6 weeks, then steady improvement, but 12 month scores were significantly lower than pretreatment ($P < 0.008$). The persistent low sexual function score was entirely responsible for the result; all other scores within the prostate cancer domain showed no significant change from baseline at 12 months. It is generally accepted that erectile dysfunction is higher after prostate cryotherapy than with other treatment modalities. In this study, of 46 potent men, only one had functional erections at 12 months. The authors note that the average time to return to work in this series was 3 weeks.

The study was updated with repeat FACT-P surveys and a Sexuality Follow-Up Questionnaire at 3 years post treatment.[5] The Sexual Follow-Up Questionnaire is a tool developed for this study and is not a validated instrument. The study reported on 75 men and showed overall stability of the previously reported 12 month outcomes.[6] The social/family well-being domain showed no further recovery in the intervening 2 years, and remained below baseline (although not statistically different) at 36 months. The Prostate Cancer Therapy specific domain did show interval improvements, and total score returned to baseline pretreatment levels. At the 12-month mark the prostate domain score was lower than baseline due to low sexual function scores. In the subsequent 2 years these scores improved and thus the total score returned to baseline. However, for most men, sexual function does not return to baseline. In the updated series, complete 3-year survey data were available on 38 subjects who had normal erections pretreatment. There were five subjects who recovered potency by year 3, with an additional 13 men able to resume sexual activity with erectile aids. This yields a sexual function rate of 47% at 3 years.

There is not a study directly comparing cryotherapy to other forms of therapy for localized prostate cancer. There are other studies of localized prostate cancer therapies which utilized the FACT tool with which general comparisons can be made. Litwin et al used the FACT-general form in their study of men who had undergone prostatectomy, pelvic irradiation, or observation for localized prostate cancer.[7] These groups were compared to an age-matched population without prostate cancer. The groups had undergone treatment or diagnosis on average 5–6 years prior to completing the survey. The scores on the general FACT domains were very similar to slightly lower than the general scores at 36 months post-cryotherapy. It should be noted that the cryotherapy group was younger (mean age 66) than the prostatectomy (mean age 69.7) or radiation (mean age 76.2) groups.

Lee et al used the FACT-P tool to follow QOL outcomes over 12 months in patients undergoing brachytherapy, external beam radiotherapy, and radical prostatectomy.[8] They used version 3 of the FACT-P, which has 34 questions in the general domain, but used the same 12 question prostate cancer treatment domain. The surveys were given pretreatment and at 1, 3, and 12 months after treatment. The median ages in the groups were 67 for brachytherapy, 68.8 for external beam radiotherapy, and 61 for radical prostatectomy. Brachytherapy showed a trend similar to cryotherapy with significantly lower prostate domain scores at 1 and 3 months, but return to near baseline at 12 months. The 12 month prostate domain score was not significantly lower than the pretreatment score for brachytherapy, whereas it did remain significantly lower for cryotherapy. External beam radiotherapy showed no statistically significant changes over the 12 months. Radical prostatectomy showed significantly lower prostate domain score at 1 month only, but returned to baseline by 12 months.

A second study of prostate cryotherapy using a validated quality-of-life questionnaire comes from Columbia University.[9] Anastasiadis et al used the European Organization for Research and Treatment of Cancer (EORTC) instrument with the prostate cancer domain supplement, to study 131 consecutive patients. The EORTC QOL instrument is a 30-question survey specifically designed to capture data on patients undergoing cancer trials. A secondary module was developed to measure prostate cancer specific treatment side effects on sexual, bowel, and urinary function. Patients were mailed the questionnaire at least 6 months post-treatment. No baseline surveys were done pretreatment. Fifty-one patients who had primary cryotherapy and 30 patients who had salvage cryotherapy returned questionnaires. As one would expect, when comparing the primary to the salvage group, the primary therapy group had better scores overall, but only the physical and social scores were significantly higher for the primary treatment group.

The authors compared scores from this study to two other published studies of radiation therapy that used the EORTC survey. The cryotherapy scores for the general health domains were equivalent to the radiation study scores.

The modern generation of cryotherapy has reduced the rate of serious complications. Smaller cryoprobes, real-time ultrasound guidance, and reliable urethral warmers have decreased rates of urethral sloughing, and rectal fistula is now quite rare. Studies using these modern systems should be used for discussing side effects.

Rates of urinary incontinence and erectile dysfunction will vary tremendously depending on the definitions used and the manner of data collection. Patient-completed questionnaires will generally yield higher rates of complications than physician reports. Table 7.1 lists some modern primary cryotherapy series and their reported side-effect rates. The definitions are also listed.

In summary, cryotherapy shows favorable quality-of-life scores at up to 3 years post-treatment. There are no appreciable late complications. Similar to radical prostatectomy and brachytherapy, there is a short-term decline in quality of life, which rapidly recovers. The majority of men will remain impotent after treatment.

Table 7.1				
	Incontinence (%)	Potent (%)	Urinary obstruction (%)	Recto-urinary fistula (%)
Long[10]	2[a]	12[c]	6[f]	0
Prepelica[11]	3[b]		3[g]	0
Han[12]	3[b]	13[d]	5[f]	0
Robinson[5,6]		6–34[e]		0

[a] Any pad use at 12 months.
[b] Any daily pad use.
[c] Intact erections noted in physician chart.
[d] Unnamed patient-reported questionnaires.
[e] FACT-P survey 6% potent at 24 months, 34% active using aids at 3 years.
[f] Urethral sloughing.
[g] Urinary retention.

There is a role for medical therapy of erectile dysfunction in this patient population. The high rate of persistent sexual dysfunction did not translate into an overall decline in health-related quality of life in this series of patients. The current generation of cryotherapy equipment has an excellent side-effect profile.

REFERENCES

1. Litwin MS, Lubeck DP, Henning JM, Carroll PR. Differences in urologist and patient assessments of health related quality of life in men with prostate cancer: results of the CaPSURE database. J Urol 1998; 159 (6): 1988–92.
2. Penson DF, Litwin MS, Aaronson NK. Health related quality of life in men with prostate cancer [see comment]. J Urol 2003; 169 (5): 1653–61.
3. Cella DF, Tulsky DS, Gray G et al. The Functional Assessment of Cancer Therapy scale: development and validation of the general measure. J Clin Oncol 1993; 11 (3): 570–9.
4. Esper P, Mo F, Chodak G et al. Measuring quality of life in men with prostate cancer using the functional assessment of cancer therapy-prostate instrument. Urology 1997; 50 (6): 920–8.
5. Robinson JW, Donnelly BJ, Saliken JC et al. Quality of life and sexuality of men with prostate cancer 3 years after cryosurgery. Urology 2002; 60 (2 Suppl 1): 12–18.
6. Robinson JW, Saliken JC, Donnelly BJ et al. Quality-of-life outcomes for men treated with cryosurgery for localized prostate carcinoma. Cancer 1999; 86 (9): 1793–801.
7. Litwin MS, Hays RD, Fink A et al. Quality-of-life outcomes in men treated for localized prostate cancer [see comment]. JAMA 1995; 273 (2): 129–35.
8. Lee WR, Hall MC, McQuellon RP et al. A prospective quality-of-life study in men with clinically localized prostate carcinoma treated with radical prostatectomy, external beam radiotherapy, or interstitial brachytherapy. Int J Radiat Oncol Biol Phys 2001; 51 (3): 614–23.
9. Anastasiadis AG, Sachdev R, Salomon L et al. Comparison of health-related quality of life and prostate-associated symptoms after primary and salvage cryotherapy for prostate cancer. J Cancer Res Clin Oncol 2003; 129 (12): 676–82.
10. Long JP, Bahn D, Lee F et al. Five-year retrospective, multi-institutional pooled analysis of cancer-related outcomes after cryosurgical ablation of the prostate. Urology 2001; 57 (3): 518–23.
11. Prepelica KL, Okeke Z, Murphy A, Katz AE. Cryosurgical ablation of the prostate: high risk patient outcomes. Cancer 2005; 103 (8): 1625–30.
12. Han KR, Belldegrun AS. Third-generation cryosurgery for primary and recurrent prostate cancer. BJU Int 2004; 93 (1): 14–18.

8

Technique of renal cryoablation

Brant R. Fulmer

Introduction • Terminology • Basic cryobiology • Cryosurgical equipment
• Indications for renal cryosurgery • Informed consent • Renal biopsy
• Technique of cryoprobe placement • Open renal cryoablation • Laparoscopic-guided renal cryoablation • Percutaneous image-guided renal cryoablation
• Percutaneous ultrasound-guided renal cryoablation • Computed tomographic guided-renal cryoablation • Magnetic resonance imaging-guided renal cryosurgery
• Conclusion

INTRODUCTION

The ideal renal cryoablative procedure has the relatively simple goal of freezing a desired lesion within the kidney to produce a predictable area of tissue death. The overall goal is to destroy a predetermined amount of tissue with a normal rim of renal parenchyma, thus recreating, as much as possible, surgical extirpation.[1] Significant and rapid advances in the technology responsible to produce rapid tissue freezing have served to improve accuracy and predictability for this technique. In addition, our understanding of cryobiology and the direct and indirect mechanisms of cryogenic tissue injury have also improved.

In order to be considered to be technically successful, a renal cryoablation procedure involves completion of three basic steps: localization of the kidney lesion, application of cryoablative energy, and complete tissue coverage by intraoperative monitoring. Although simple to describe, this chapter outlines some of the challenges that are faced performing this kind of tissue ablation.

TERMINOLOGY

In the science of tissue ablation, communicating with universally accepted terminology is essential to allow for precise descriptions of technique and accurate result reporting. A recent report from the radiology-sponsored International Working Group on Image-Guided Tumor Ablation provides the first organized effort in standardizing the terminology and reporting criteria for tissue ablation.[2,3] The pertinent terms as they relate to renal cryosurgery are used in the text of this chapter, and are available for review and reference in Appendix 1.

BASIC CRYOBIOLOGY

Cryogenic injury to tissue can be divided into both direct and indirect effects. The immediate direct effect of rapidly cooling tissue is extracellular compartment freezing followed by intracellular ice crystal formation resulting in cellular membrane disruption.[1,4] This type of injury kills cells directly and results in a predictable area of coagulative necrosis. The indirect effects include microcirculatory ischemia which occurs during the thawing phase.[5] There is also microvascular hemorrhage noted beyond the margin of the ablated lesion.[6] The thermal ablation zone then undergoes a series of steps including fibrosis, scarring, and collagen deposition. Several studies have confirmed the necessity of achieving temperatures of −20°C to achieve permanent tissue damage and most authors use −40°C as the temperature to achieve lethal iceball formation.[4,7,8]

This conservative approach using the −40°C isotherm allows for an adequate ablation margin with the overlap of the −20°C isotherm that is also typically lethal.

Several studies have shown that two freeze cycles are necessary to provide reproducible cell death in the desired cryoablation zone as dictated by the −20°C to −40°C isotherms,[9,10] but active vs. passive thawing once represented a significant controversy in the field of tissue cryoablation. Most studies demonstrate no difference comparing active and passive thawing,[10,11] and it is the opinion of most ablationists that active thawing does not result in a decreased in technical efficacy of the procedure.[5] It does, however, reduce procedure time and results in decreased anesthesia time for the patient.[12] Perhaps, a more important concept is that of "thermal history" or the time–temperature relationship of any given tissue during an ablation procedure. If the appropriate thermal history is present, it is likely that there will be a predictable and reproducible zone of tissue necrosis following cryoablation.[12,13]

With a working knowledge of the biology of renal cryosurgical injury, the essential features of a technically successful cryoablation become readily apparent. These steps include rapid monitored freezing, passive or active thawing, and then a repeat of this cycle to achieve coverage of the planned thermal ablation zone.[5]

A note here is warranted regarding the potential effect of including a portion of the renal collecting system in the ablation zone. Several studies have reported data to suggest that the collecting system is very resistant to cryogenic injury, even with direct puncture, and will re-epithelialize following cryoablative damage to the urothelium.[14,15]

CRYOSURGICAL EQUIPMENT

The initial technology for performing cryoablation was introduced in 1992 and was based on a liquid nitrogen source for freezing. The modern gas-based cryoablative systems were introduced in 1995, and typically use argon gas for freezing with helium for active thawing. The currently available technology for renal cryosurgery comes from essentially two commercial sources. The Cryocare CS system is manufactured by Endocare, Inc., Irvine, CA, and the IceRod, SeedNet, and IceBulb systems are manufactured by Oncura, Inc., Plymouth Meeting, PA.

A representative example of a renal cryosurgical generator and console is shown in Figure 8.1. This console is coupled to tanks supplying the argon and helium gas. The cryoablative energy is applied through several varieties of commercially available cryoprobes. Each probe has a different-sized ablative zone corresponding to temperature regions called isotherms. Figures 8.2 and 8.3 demonstrate the currently available renal cryoablation probes and their corresponding isotherms from Oncura, Inc., and Endocare, Inc., respectively.

Cryoprobe size is fixed at 1.47 mm (17 gauge) in the Oncura system with maximal lethal iceball size at the −40°C isotherm of 1.45 cm × 3.4 cm. Therefore, to achieve a cryogenic ablative zone of larger that 1.45 cm, more that one probe must be used.

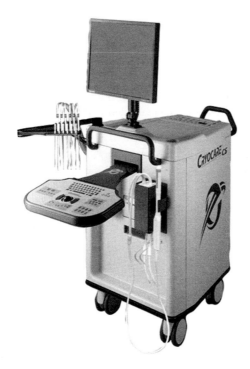

Figure 8.1 Representative example of a renal cryoablation system (courtesy of Endocare, Inc., Irvine, CA).

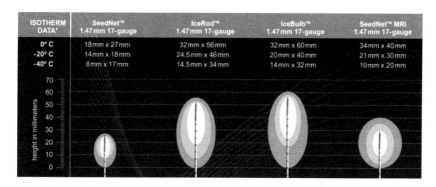

ISOTHERM DATA*	SeedNet™ 1.47 mm 17-gauge	IceRod™ 1.47 mm 17-gauge	IceBulb™ 1.47 mm 17-gauge	SeedNet™ MRI 1.47 mm 17-gauge
0° C	18 mm x 27 mm	32 mm x 56 mm	32 mm x 60 mm	34 mm x 40 mm
-20° C	14 mm x 18 mm	24.5 mm x 46 mm	20 mm x 40 mm	21 mm x 30 mm
-40° C	8 mm x 17 mm	14.5 mm x 34 mm	14 mm x 32 mm	10 mm x 20 mm

Figure 8.2 Representative Oncura, Inc. Renal cryoablation probes and isotherms (courtesy of Oncura, Inc., Plymouth Meeting, PA).

The Endocare system has cryoprobes ranging in diameter from 1.7 to 3.8 mm, with maximal lethal iceball size at the −40°C isotherm of 2.4 cm × 4.4 cm for the largest probe (3.8 mm). The maximal lethal iceball for the Endocare 1.7 mm probe is 1.4 cm × 3.5 cm. As will be discussed later, it is an important observation that the lethal iceball does not extend appreciably from the tip of the cryoprobe, thus necessitating careful placement of the cryoprobe tip at or just past the deep margin of the lesion to be ablated.

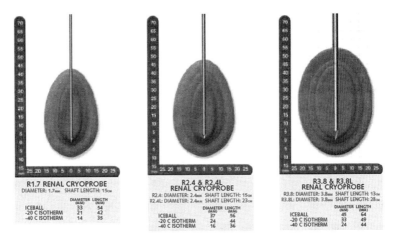

Figure 8.3 Representative Endocare, Inc. Renal cryoablation probes and isotherms (courtesy of Endocare, Inc., Irvine, CA).

Another consideration in using the cryoablation system is that it is difficult to measure temperature in the tissue at the site of thermal ablation. Both of the commercially available cryosurgical systems measure the temperature of the gas in the probe as a surrogate for direct measurement of the temperature at the probe tip. This temperature correlates indirectly with the expected isotherms in that achieving temperatures of $-180°C$ to $-200°C$ will yield a lethal $-40°C$ isotherm in the expected distribution for that probe. The only way to measure temperature in the surrounding tissue is to place the available thermocouple temperature probes in the tissue at the area that temperature measurement is desired, and continuously measure during the course of the ablation.

INDICATIONS FOR RENAL CRYOSURGERY

The indications for treating a renal lesion with cryoablation are largely dependent upon the limitations for an adequate cryogenic ablation zone posed by the current technology. The larger the renal lesion, the more difficult it becomes to assure complete coverage of the lesion with the currently available cryoprobes. Although series do report large lesions treated with this technology,[16] most authors suggest that cryoablation is indicated for renal lesions less than 4.0 cm,[17–19] and some authors suggest 3.0 cm as the cutoff to assure technical success.[20]

Other potential indications include renal insufficiency, solitary kidney, renal transplant, multiple or bilateral renal masses. Patient preference also plays a substantial role in influencing choice of treatment, and the minimally invasive nature of renal cryoablation certainly makes this modality an attractive choice for properly chosen renal lesions.

INFORMED CONSENT

The technique of renal cryosurgery carries a degree of complexity even for experienced clinicians. Therefore, achieving adequate informed consent for patients can be a daunting task. We have assumed a posture of education in approaching patients with this treatment. Patients should understand that the most definitive treatment for renal cell carcinoma is still radical nephrectomy. Minimally invasive therapies seek to reproduce the clinical results of surgical extirpation, but may inherently trade some of the certainty that accompanies surgical treatment. Renal cryosurgery is a technique that spares renal functional loss while attempting to reproduce the clinical success with surgical excision. Since there is no permanent pathologic specimen, a measure of uncertainty is the trade off for the decreased morbidity of the procedure and the preservation of renal function. This point is further emphasized later in the discussion of preablation renal biopsy.

Informed consent must include a discussion of both the cryosurgical technique as well as the data available about the outcomes of renal cryosurgery. Adequate informed consent facilitates later discussions of treatment outcome as well as the possible need for retreatment.

RENAL BIOPSY

Improvements in the technology of renal imaging have resulted in being able to identify malignant renal lesions with cross-sectional imaging with a high predictive value. Therefore, in conventional oncologic practice, biopsy of renal lesions is rarely indicated prior to definitive surgical treatment. In this setting, the specimen is typically available for pathologic analysis, thus confirming the diagnosis of malignancy and allowing accurate pathologic staging. In the setting of renal cryotherapy, however, a final pathologic specimen is not obtained, and it is routine to biopsy the renal mass to be treated. The rationale for performing a renal biopsy is that it might be useful in determining the need for observation or retreatment. An example might be a solid renal mass that is determined on core biopsy to be an oncocytoma. In this case, observation might be substituted for retreatment based on the pathology of the lesion.

The difficulty with renal biopsy comes in equivocal lesions in which the biopsy is either negative or non-diagnostic for malignancy. Given the intent of renal cryoablation, it is not necessary to send the renal biopsy for frozen section analysis. Therefore, the lesion has usually already been treated with technical success, and the biopsy report is obtained later on permanent sectioning. A non-diagnostic biopsy, therefore, has little utility, but a biopsy diagnostic for malignancy may be able to impact future care. The issue of renal biopsy is inherently complex, and must be explained as part of the informed consent process as noted above.

Renal biopsy can be performed via fine needle aspiration or core biopsy. Since the biopsy is typically done at the time of definitive therapy, core biopsy is recommended. Image guidance allows direct and accurate placement of the biopsy gun needle in order to maximize tissue yield. Some authors also advocate the use of a vascular access sheath to assure accurate biopsy sampling and provide the potential benefit of limiting the risk of tract seeding with multiple passes of the biopsy needle.[21]

TECHNIQUE OF CRYOPROBE PLACEMENT

There is a paucity of published data regarding the specific technique for placing renal cryoprobes. Several strategies exist to assure cryoprobe placement that provides adequate coverage for renal lesion while maximally conserving normal renal parenchyma. Although most image-guided techniques allow real-time monitoring

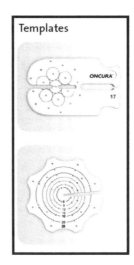

Figure 8.4 Templates for percutaneous placement of cryoprobes (courtesy of Oncura, Inc., Plymouth Meeting, PA).

of the cryoablative procedure, the size of the iceball in its entirety does not represent a lethal thermal ablative zone. Therefore, a thorough knowledge of the renal cryoprobe configuration and isotherms is necessary for the accurate placement of probes prior to beginning the freezing process.

As previously elucidated, one of the most important technical concepts involves placement of the cryoprobe tip at or slightly beyond the deep margin of the lesion to be treated. If this is not performed in a precise manner, the lesion may be incompletely treated due to the small amount of lethal ice at the tip of the cryoprobe. Once this has been accomplished, adequate coverage of the renal lesion simply involves placement of enough probes to cover the longitudinal diameter of the lesion.

Since most of the image-guidance technology used for probe placement has the capacity for measurement, one technique for assuring adequate cryoablative coverage is to position all probes so that no margin of the tumor is more than the distance of the radius of the lethal iceball away from any given probe. This is sometimes difficult due to the three-dimensional configuration of the renal lesion. The use of a template (Figure 8.4) may be beneficial to evenly space the cryoprobes and overlap lethal cryoablative zones to assure adequate coverage. Templates are particularly useful when using multiple small cryoprobes. Some of the cryoablative systems allow the operator to partially freeze a probe to hold it in position. This technique is very useful in the case of a highly mobile kidney or in a kidney where probes are to be placed in several different planes to conform to the three-dimensional orientation of the renal lesion.

Another useful technique is the use of temperature probes for real-time monitoring of the cryoablation zone. Cryoablation probes are placed as noted above and then temperature probes are placed at or just beyond the periphery of the lesion. During the active freezing process, these temperature probes can be used to assess that an adequate thermal ablative margin is achieved. The goal would be to provide lethal ice about 0.5–1.0 cm beyond the edge of the lesion, thus assuring complete necrosis. Temperature probes can be used in difficult cases where the presence of large blood vessels may cause perfusion-mediated tissue heating, thus making the thermoablative defect less complete. Temperature probes can also be used for monitoring the temperatures in adjacent organs.

OPEN RENAL CRYOABLATION

Open renal cryoablation is perhaps the simplest technique to apply cryogenic thermal energy to a renal lesion.[22–24] The advantages of this technique include excellent visualization and tactile feedback for cryoprobe placement. Disadvantages include the large incision typically required for renal exposure resulting in a prolonged postoperative recovery. Difficulty with retreatment also exists as repeat renal exposure is more difficult in a previously operated field.

Once the lesion is identified and characterized preoperatively on imaging, the patient is given general anesthesia and an appropriate incision is made to allow exposure of the area of the kidney containing the lesion. Using a conventional hand-held probe, ultrasound mapping of the kidney can be performed, and the lesion can be characterized and measured. Ultrasound is also used to rule out multifocal disease. The predetermined number of cryoprobes is then placed using ultrasonographic guidance and the cryoablation can be monitored in real time to assure adequate coverage of the renal lesion. This technique for application of cryoablation enjoys the longest follow-up, with studies potentially providing data approaching 10 years maturity.[23]

LAPAROSCOPIC-GUIDED RENAL CRYOABLATION

The most widely described method for performing renal cryoablation is using laparoscopic guidance.[9,19,25–30] Laparoscopic access is obtained either via a transperitoneal or retroperitoneal approach. The transperitoneal approach is ideal for anterior renal lesions and gives reasonable access to the entire anterior surface of the kidney. It necessarily involves some exposure of the kidney via incision of the peritoneal reflection on the right and the line of Toldt with colon reflection on the left. The retroperitoneal approach requires balloon dissection and insufflation of the retroperitoneal space posterior and lateral to the kidney. This approach provides excellent exposure for posterior and lateral renal lesions but is a less familiar view to most urologists. It is usually employed in large measure by only more experienced laparoscopic surgeons.[19,31] Regardless of the laparoscopic approach employed, the surgeon typically performs the minimal exposure required to allow adequate visualization of the renal lesion.

Once the kidney is exposed, a laparoscopic, articulating ultrasound probe is employed to survey the kidney and target the lesion for ablation. There is some controversy over the treatment of the renal fat overlying the lesion. In the case of exophytic lesions, the overlying renal fat can be removed and sent for frozen section or frozen *in situ* with the renal lesion. For endophytic or central lesions, the perirenal fat is left intact. When the lesion is adequately visualized either directly or under ultrasound guidance, the cryoprobes are then placed under direct visualization either percutaneously or through one of the existing laparoscopic trocars. Laparoscopic technique allows direct visual puncture of the lesion, and ultrasound guidance allows excellent visualization of the deep margin for cryoprobe placement.

Visualizing renal cryoablation

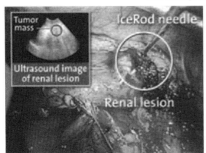
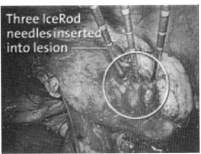

1. Identify the lesion   2. Cryoablation needles placed inside the lesion

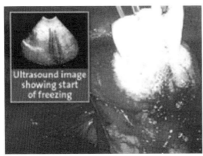
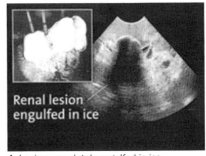

3. Monitoring iceball growth with real-time   4. Lesion completely engulfed in ice
   ultrasound guidance

Figure 8.5   Step-by-step illustration of laparoscopic renal cryoablation with ultrasound correlation (courtesy of Oncura, Inc., Plymouth Meeting, PA). (See also color plate.)

Using the previously described freezing techniques, the lesion is then cryoablated with two freeze cycles of 10–15 minutes with active thawing. A diagrammatic representation of these steps can be seen in Figure 8.5.

PERCUTANEOUS IMAGE-GUIDED RENAL CRYOABLATION

The ideal renal cryoablative procedure should naturally evolve toward the technique that provides the best balance of efficacy and decreased morbidity. As a minimally invasive technique, percutaneous renal cryoablation holds perhaps the greatest promise at providing this desired combination. The advantages of percutaneous renal cryoablation are clear. The less-invasive nature of this procedure provides the patient with decreased morbidity and faster recovery. Moreover, it has been noted that percutaneous renal cryoablation carries a lower perioperative analgesic requirement compared to other ablative technologies like radiofrequency ablation or laparoscopy.[32]

   In general, all variations of renal cryoablation technique employ the use of imaging modalities for preoperative planning and treatment monitoring. As the technique of renal cryoablation procedure becomes less invasive, the utilization and reliance on sophisticated imaging modalities increases. Using the terminology of the International Working Group on Image-Guided Tumor Ablation, diagnostic imaging modalities are commonly used for several functions during an ablative procedure. Initial diagnosis, staging, and planning of treatment for the lesion begin the process.

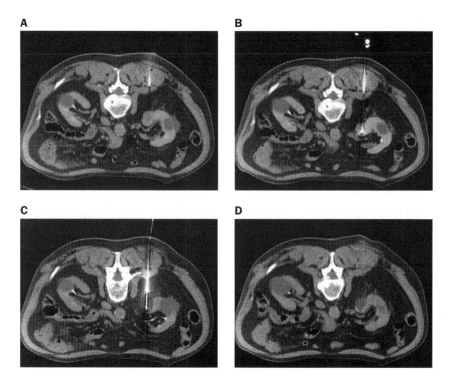

Figure 8.6 Step-by-step illustration of CT-guided cryoablation. (A) Pretreatment view of the posterior 1.5×2.0 cm solid renal mass. (B) Cryoprobe placement with needle tip at the deep margin of tumor. (C) Mature iceball formation noted by decreased tissue density in area of previous renal lesion. (D) Post-ablation image showing treated zone of necrosis.

Image guidance is then used for targeting, monitoring, and controlling the actual cryoablative procedure. Postoperative imaging with CT scan or MRI is the mainstay for assessing treatment response following ablative treatment.[3]

In general, percutaneous renal cryoablation is performed using ultrasound, CT, or MRI guidance. Each technique has advantages and disadvantages compared to other techniques, but each employs the same basic steps to achieve an adequate zone of cryoablation. Further, each technique requires a different set of skills and may necessarily require the participation of a urologist, radiologist, or both to assure technical success. The techniques are described individually as follows.

PERCUTANEOUS ULTRASOUND-GUIDED RENAL CRYOABLATION

Ultrasound guidance for percutaneous renal cryoablation was first described in the literature in 2004.[33] Ultrasound guidance has several advantages for the placement of renal cryoprobes and also the monitoring of the ablative procedure. A defined pattern of changes on ultrasound during tissue freezing coupled with minimal radiation exposure makes this technique ideal for real-time monitoring of cryoablative treatment. Tissue changes during freezing include early development of a hyperechoic rim around the lesion followed by the hypoechoic iceball formation.[34] Representative ultrasound pictures can be seen in Figure 8.6.

Ultrasound is ideal for lateral and lower-pole exophytic lesions. Upper-pole and posterior lesions represent a more difficult challenge due to the difficulty imaging the kidney through the overlying ribs. Endophytic lesions can also be treated by this method; small lesions may be difficult to visualize depending on the experience of the ultrasound operator. These procedures are commonly performed with the assistance of a radiologist or ultrasound technician. At many centers such as ours, percutaneous renal cryoablation is performed with the urologist solely performing and interpreting the ultrasound. Our technique is described briefly as follows.

In brief, the patient is placed in a full flank lateral decubitus position after the induction of MAC or general anesthesia. Initial planning and targeting of the lesion is performed by surveying the kidney and imaging the lesion in several planes. Measurements are taken of the mass and compared to preoperative cross-sectional imaging. Plane of entry and trajectory of the cryoprobes is then determined by using the biopsy guide on the percutaneous renal ultrasound probe. Once the cryoprobe(s) placement is planned, the biopsy guide is then used to perform core biopsy needle using a prostate biopsy gun. The first of the percutaneous biopsy probes is then placed using the biopsy guide. Care is taken to avoid medial placement of the cryoprobes to minimize risk of bowel injury. The cryoprobe is advanced to the posterior margin of the mass by real-time ultrasound monitoring. If necessary, additional cryoprobes are placed using either a premeasured percutaneous template or with the use of the ultrasound probe biopsy guide. It is sometimes necessary to change the trajectory of the cryoprobe in order to assure thermal ablation zone coverage of irregular lesions. The cryoablation is then performed using two 10–15 minute freeze cycles with active thawing. Real-time ultrasound monitoring of the ablation is performed throughout the freezing process. Additional cryoprobe placement or repositioning is performed if there is evidence of incomplete ablative coverage of the lesion.

Overall, there is a paucity of data regarding long-term follow-up of percutaneous ultrasound-guided renal cryoablation. With increased utilization, mature data series are anticipated.

COMPUTED TOMOGRAPHIC-GUIDED RENAL CRYOABLATION

The routine use of CT scanning in the diagnosis and staging of renal tumors makes CT guidance an obvious choice for performing image-guided renal cryoablation. Direct correlation to the preoperative imaging is possible and multifocality of disease is easily assessed. In addition, CT guidance allows for very precise cryoprobe placement and real-time monitoring of therapy. In addition, recent reports suggest that CT-guided renal cryotherapy can be successfully performed using conscious sedation,[35] although most institutions still use general anesthesia.

Two different CT modalities are commonly used for both cryoprobe placement and monitoring. CT scan images can either be obtained using spiral CT technology or CT-guided fluoroscopy. For spiral CT-guided cryoablation, the lesion is mapped and using anatomic landmarks and distance to the renal lesion, the initial renal cryoprobe is advanced percutaneously. Several additional runs of spiral CT may be necessary to achieve adequate positioning of the renal cryoprobe. The advantage of a sheath for renal biopsy is apparent here to reduce the overall radiation dose to the patient that might be required for multiple passes of the biopsy needle. In contradistinction, CT-guided fluoroscopy allows for real-time insertion and positioning of cryoprobes into the renal lesion. The tradeoff is a much higher radiation dose to the radiologist or urologist.

Once the cryoprobes are placed, the ablative technique is then identical to that previously described with two 10–15-minute cycles with active thawing. CT characteristics of the cryoablative zone were first described over 20 years ago,[36] and include decreases in the density of the tissue on CT scan with cooling that are most pronounced with change in phase from iceball formation. Modern studies confirm the routine use of CT guidance for real-time monitoring of renal cryoablation.[18,37] Much like ultrasound, measurement of the iceball on CT is a primary determinant of adequate coverage of the cryoablation zone. A representative example of a percutaneous renal cryoablation of a posterior renal lesion is shown in Figure 8.6.

MAGNETIC RESONANCE IMAGING-GUIDED RENAL CRYOSURGERY

Magnetic resonance imaging provides equal or increased accuracy compared to CT scan, and has the added advantage of not exposing the patient to high levels of radiation. These advantages have served to make this the modality of choice in many centers for percutaneous-guided renal cryoablation. Disadvantages of MRI guidance include increased cost as well as the availability of an open or operative MRI system. Some patients may also have contraindications to MRI including pacemakers, implants, etc. Finally, MRI technology is less familiar to most urologists and usually requires collaboration with radiology.

MRI changes during freezing are due to the very short T2 relaxation time of ice that affords excellent contrast between the ice and surrounding tissue, allowing an accurate depiction of the entire extent of the iceball. The iceball presents visually as a sharply marginated region of signal loss that expands and engulfs the renal lesion with clear contrast to surrounding tissue.[38]

Essential steps to performing MRI-guided renal cryoablation are similar to CT-guided ablation and include planning and targeting with MRI guidance, real-time or staged placement of cryoprobes, and two 10–15-minute freeze cycles with active thawing. MRI has been reported for use in cases of solitary kidney, multiple renal lesions, and transplant kidneys.[16,39,40] MRI, like CT scan, is also an ideal modality for image-guided cryoablation of central or endophytic renal lesions.

There is minimal reported long-term data regarding the efficacy of renal cryoablation performed under MRI guidance. Moreover, even the largest series consist of only 10–20 patients.[41–43] We will anxiously await the 5-year long-term outcome data of this technique.

CONCLUSION

This chapter has sought to outline the basic technique of renal cryoablation, and to describe the many variations on the common procedural theme. Regardless of modality, the basic goal of renal cryosurgery remains to accurately and reliably reproduce a lethal cryoablative zone that results in a predictable area of tissue death. The literature suggests that image-guided renal cryoablation done by any technique can provide both immediate technical success as well as demonstrating technical effectiveness in short-term follow-up. Updated data from early cryoablation series are needed to start to evaluate the long-term efficacy and durability of this procedure.

REFERENCES

1. Gill IS, Novick AC. Renal cryosurgery. Urology 1999; 54 (2): 215–19.
2. Goldberg SN, Charboneau JW, Dodd GD et al. Image-guided tumor ablation: proposal for standardization of terms and reporting criteria. Radiology 2003; 228 (2): 335–45.
3. Goldberg SN, Grassi CJ, Cardella JF et al. Image-guided tumor ablation: standardization of terminology and reporting criteria. Radiology 2005; 16 (6): 765–78.
4. Chosy SG, Nakada SY, Lee FT Jr, Warner TF. Monitoring renal cryosurgery: predictors of tissue necrosis in swine. J Urol 1998; 159 (4): 1370–4.
5. Gill IS. Minimally invasive nephron-sparing surgery. Urol Clin North Am 2003; 30 (3): 551–79.
6. Edmunds TB Jr, Schulsinger DA, Durand DB, Waltzer WC. Acute histologic changes in human renal tumors after cryoablation. J Endourol 2000; 14 (2): 139–43.
7. Barone GW, Rodgers BM. Morphologic and functional effects of renal cryoinjury. Cryobiology 1988; 25 (4): 363–71.
8. Baust JG, Gage AA. The molecular basis of cryosurgery. BJU Int 2005; 95 (9): 1187–91.
9. Bishoff JT, Chen RB, Lee BR et al. Laparoscopic renal cryoablation: acute and long-term clinical, radiographic, and pathologic effects in an animal model and application in a clinical trial. J Endourol 1999; 13 (4): 233–9.
10. Woolley ML, Schulsinger DA, Durand DB et al. Effect of freezing parameters (freeze cycle and thaw process) on tissue destruction following renal cryoablation. J Endourol 2002; 16 (7): 519–22.
11. Finelli A, Rewcastle JC, Jewett MA. Cryotherapy and radiofrequency ablation: pathophysiologic basis and laboratory studies. Curr Opin Urol 2003; 13 (3): 187–91.
12. Hoffmann NE, Bischof JC. The cryobiology of cryosurgical injury. Urology 2002; 60 (2 Suppl 1): 40–9.
13. Rupp CC, Hoffmann NE, Schmidlin FR et al. Cryosurgical changes in the porcine kidney: histologic analysis with thermal history correlation. Cryobiology 2002; 45 (2): 167–82.
14. Janzen NK, Perry KT, Han KR et al. The effects of intentional cryoablation and radio frequency ablation of renal tissue involving the collecting system in a porcine model. J Urol 2005; 173 (4): 1368–74.
15. Sung GT, Gill IS, Hsu T et al. Effect of intentional cryo-injury to the renal collecting system. J Urol 2003; 170 (2 Pt 1): 619–22.
16. Shingleton WB, Sewell PE Jr. Percutaneous renal cryoablation of renal tumors in patients with von Hippel–Lindau disease. J Urol 2002; 167 (3): 1268–70.
17. Powell T, Whelan C, Schwartz BF. Laparoscopic renal cryotherapy: biology, techniques and outcomes. Minerva Urol Nefrol 2005; 57 (2): 109–18.
18. Pareek G, Nakada SY. The current role of cryotherapy for renal and prostate tumors. Urol Oncol 2005; 23 (5): 361–6.
19. Gill IS, Remer EM, Hasan WA et al. Renal cryoablation: outcome at 3 years. J Urol 2005; 173 (6): 1903–7.
20. Spaliviero M, Moinzadeh A, Gill IS. Laparoscopic cryotherapy for renal tumors. Technol Cancer Res Treat 2004; 3 (2): 177–80.
21. Rapp DE, Orvieto M, Sokoloff MH, Shalhav AL. Use of biopsy sheath to improve standardization of renal mass biopsy in tissue-ablative procedures. J Endourol 2004; 18 (5): 453–4.
22. Pantuck AJ, Zisman A, Cohen J, Belldegrun A. Cryosurgical ablation of renal tumors using 1.5-millimeter, ultrathin cryoprobes. Urology 2002; 59 (1): 130–3.
23. Rukstalis DB, Khorsandi M, Garcia FU et al. Clinical experience with open renal cryoablation. Urology 2001; 57 (1): 34–9.
24. Zegel HG, Holland GA, Jennings SB et al. Intraoperative ultrasonographically guided cryoablation of renal masses: initial experience. J Ultrasound Med 1998; 17 (9): 571–6.
25. Cestari A, Guazzoni G, dell'Acqua V et al. Laparoscopic cryoablation of solid renal masses: intermediate term follow-up. J Urol 2004; 172 (4 Pt 1): 1267–70.
26. Chen RN, Novick AC, Gill IS. Laparoscopic cryoablation of renal masses. Urol Clin North Am 2000; 27 (4): 813–20.

27. Gill IS, Novick AC, Meraney AM et al. Laparoscopic renal cryoablation in 32 patients. Urology 2000; 56 (5): 748–53.
28. Johnson DB, Nakada SY. Laparoscopic cryoablation for renal-cell cancer. J Endourol 2000; 14 (10): 873–8; discussion 878–9.
29. Moon TD, Lee FT Jr, Hedican SP et al. Laparoscopic cryoablation under sonographic guidance for the treatment of small renal tumors. J Endourol 2004; 18 (5): 436–40.
30. Nadler RB, Kim SC, Rubenstein JN et al. Laparoscopic renal cryosurgery: the Northwestern experience. J Urol 2003; 170 (4 Pt 1): 1121–5.
31. Lee DI, McGinnis DE, Feld R, Strup SE. Retroperitoneal laparoscopic cryoablation of small renal tumors: intermediate results. Urology 2003; 61 (1): 83–8.
32. Allaf ME, Varkarakis IM, Bhayani SB et al. Pain control requirements for percutaneous ablation of renal tumors: cryoablation versus radiofrequency ablation – initial observations. Radiology 2005; 237 (1): 366–70.
33. Bassignani MJ, Moore Y, Watson L, Theodorescu D. Pilot experience with real-time ultrasound guided percutaneous renal mass cryoablation. J Urol 2004; 171 (4): 1620–3.
34. Onik GM, Reyes G, Cohen JK, Porterfield B. Ultrasound characteristics of renal cryosurgery. Urology 1993; 42 (2): 212–15.
35. Gupta A, Allaf ME, Kavoussi LR et al. Computerized tomography guided percutaneous renal cryoablation with the patient under conscious sedation: initial clinical experience. J Urol 2006; 175 (2): 447–52; discussion 452–3.
36. Reiser M, Drukier AK, Ultsch B, Feuerbach S. The use of CT in monitoring cryosurgery. Eur J Radiol 1983; 3 (2): 123–8.
37. Lee DI, Clayman RV. Percutaneous approaches to renal cryoablation. J Endourol 2004; 18 (7): 643–6.
38. Harada J, Mogami T. Minimally invasive therapy under image guidance – emphasizing MRI-guided cryotherapy. Rinsho Byori 2004; 52 (2): 145–51.
39. Shingleton WB, Sewell PE. Percutaneous cryoablation of renal cell carcinoma in a transplanted kidney. BJU Int 2002; 90 (1): 137–8.
40. Shingleton WB, Sewell PE Jr. Cryoablation of renal tumours in patients with solitary kidneys. BJU Int 2003; 92 (3): 237–9.
41. Harada J, Dohi M, Mogami T et al. Initial experience of percutaneous renal cryosurgery under the guidance of a horizontal open MRI system. Radiat Med 2001; 19 (6): 291–6.
42. Shingleton WB, Sewell PE Jr. Percutaneous renal tumor cryoablation with magnetic resonance imaging guidance. J Urol 2001 165 (3): 773–6.
43. Silverman SG, Tuncali K, van Sonnenberg E et al. Renal tumors: MR imaging-guided percutaneous cryotherapy – initial experience in 23 patients. Radiology 2005; 236 (2): 716–24.

APPENDIX 1: STANDARD TERMINOLOGY FOR RENAL CRYOSURGICAL PROCEDURES*

Cryoablation/cryotherapy – describe all methods of destroying tissue that involve application of low-temperature freezing.

Cryoprobe – applicator for cold thermal energy.

Heat sink effect – alteration in the shape of the thermal ablation zone away from a visible, >1 mm blood vessel due to the undesired addition of heat.

*Adapted from Goldberg SN, Grassi CJ, Cardella JF et al; Society of Interventional Radiology, Technology Assessment Committee; International Working Group on Image-Guided Tumor Ablation. Image guided tumor ablation: standardization of terminology and results reporting. Radiology, 2005; 235 (3): 728–39.

Perfusion-mediated tissue heating – refers both the heat sink effect as well as the contribution of capillary microperfusion which can alter the shape and size of the thermal ablation zone.

Primary effectiveness rate – percentage of tumors effectively ablated following initial treatment or defined course of therapy.

Secondary or assisted effectiveness rate – includes tumors that are ablated after more than one treatment, or those that require retreatment after local progression.

Technical success – was the tumor treated according to protocol – immediate.

Technique effectiveness – was the tumor successfully ablated – delayed.

Thermal ablation – destruction of tumor using the application of thermal energy; application of heat (RF) or cold (cryosurgery) both constitute thermal ablative therapies.

9

Renal cryoablation: clinical outcomes

John S. Lam, Peter G. Schulam, Arie S. Belldegrun

INTRODUCTION

Over 36 000 new cases of renal cell carcinoma (RCC) are diagnosed annually and more than 12 000 deaths occur from this disease each year in the United States.[1] Radical nephrectomy has been the gold standard for the management of renal tumors since Robson and colleagues reported greater survival in patients who underwent this procedure compared those who underwent simple nephrectomy.[2] However, widespread use of abdominal computed tomography (CT), ultrasound, and magnetic resonance imaging (MRI) has led to an increased detection of incidental and relatively small renal masses. Approaches to managing small renal masses have evolved in the last two decades. Indications for nephron-sparing surgery have expanded, and minimally invasive procedures, which can confer advantages over open surgery, are now available. Ablative techniques offer a combination of nephron-sparing and minimally invasive approaches. Watchful waiting in selected cases is occasionally offered as an option, based on data suggesting that small lesions (<3 cm) are slow-growing and may not pose a risk for progression and dissemination.[3–6] Ablative techniques include cryoablation, radiofrequency ablation (RFA), and high-intensity focused ultrasound. Ablative techniques require long-term studies to confirm lasting efficacy. The best modality for tumor targeting, monitoring of therapy, and follow-up remains under investigation.

NEPHRON-SPARING SURGERY WITH NORMAL CONTRALATERAL KIDNEY

Prior to the extensive use of CT and other imaging modalities, RCCs less than 3 cm in diameter accounted for approximately 5% of cases.[7] Currently, 10–40% of renal tumors are discovered when less than 3 cm in size. Reluctance to perform radical nephrectomy for small bilateral tumors or small unilateral tumors in patients with a solitary kidney and/or compromised renal function led to the development of nephron-sparing surgery.[8,9] Over time, the indication for nephron-sparing surgery has been extended to include patients with a renal mass and a normally functioning contralateral kidney.[10,11] Large series studies have confirmed similar 5-year cancer-specific survival rates between partial and radical nephrectomy.[11–15] Local recurrence rates in patients treated with partial nephrectomy have ranged between 2 and 6%.[12,14,16] Furthermore, although elective partial nephrectomy is generally performed in patients with tumors ≤4 cm, there are emerging data that partial nephrectomy can be performed on patients with larger tumors that are anatomically amenable, provided an adequate surgical margin can be safely obtained.[17,18]

RENAL CRYOBIOLOGY

The mechanisms of cryoablative cell injury and death, including the factors affecting tissue destruction, have been previously discussed in this book. This section will briefly focus on cryobiology specific to renal cryoablation. Uchida and colleagues[19] froze renal cancer cell lines for 60 minutes at $-5°C$ to $-30°C$ and found that 96% of RCC cells survived when cooled to above $-10°C$, whereas only 15% survived when cooled to below $-20°C$. Experimental and clinical reports in the treatment of non-urological malignancies show that tissue temperatures as low as $-40°C$ to $-50°C$ are required to induce complete cell death.[20] Therefore, adequate margins should be obtained by proper location of the $-40°C$ isotherm at the tumor margin. Campbell and co-workers[21] correlated intrarenal temperatures with the sonographic appearance of the cryolesion created with 3.4-mm cryoprobes in mongrel dogs and found that the iceball needed to extend at least 3.1 mm beyond the sonographic edge of the tumor to ensure adequate cooling of the tissue to at least $-20°C$. Gill and associates[22] routinely extend the iceball 1 cm beyond the tumor edge.

Some investigators have speculated on the possibility of achieving lower tissue temperatures by occluding the renal artery during cryoablation. Collyer and co-workers[23] evaluated the effects of renal vascular control and intrarenal cooling (retrograde intracavitary ice-cold saline perfusion) on the size of renal lesions attainable with a single 3.4-mm cryoprobe in a porcine model. There was no statistically significant difference found between the lesions produced acutely with renal hilar clamping alone (37.6 mm) and clamping plus intrarenal cooling (40.4 mm); however, both were significantly larger than the control cryolesions (28.7 mm). At 1 week, the area of complete necrosis produced with clamping plus intrarenal cooling (34.3 mm) was significantly larger than the areas of necrosis produced by clamping alone (27.8 mm) or conventional cryoablation (23.9 mm; alpha = 0.05, Tukey's honestly significantly different [HSD] test). However, Campbell and associates[21] could not demonstrate a practical advantage of renal artery occlusion in a canine model, which resulted in no differences in the rate of cooling, nadir temperature achieved, or mean diameter of the cryoinfarcted zone. Most investigators advocate a double freeze–thaw cycle in order to ensure adequate cell death in renal tissue due to evidence for increased cytotoxicity in prostate and hepatocellular carcinoma. No direct comparison of single versus repeat freeze–thaw cycles in the treatment of RCC has been published yet.

The gross and microscopic appearance of cryoablated renal tissue has been studied in a canine model.[24] Four hours following treatment, the tissue is grossly hemorrhagic with a sharp demarcation between treated and untreated tissue, corresponding to vascular congestion, intratubular and interstitial hemorrhage, and early nuclear pyknosis. At 8 days, a central region of coagulative necrosis and a 2-mm-thick area of sublethal injury are evident; at 3 months, the region of necrosis is absorbed, and a 1–1.5-mm-thick fibrosis layer corresponds to the area of sublethal injury. Untreated tissue remains normal both in the ipsilateral and contralateral kidneys. The above findings have also been well studied and confirmed in porcine models.[25–28] Cryoinjury of the collecting system with the iceball in the absence of a physical puncture with the cryoprobe tip does not seem to result in urinary extravasation. In a porcine study with 3-month follow-up, Sung and colleagues[29] demonstrated that healing of the cryoinjured urothelium and adjacent parenchyma occurred by secondary intention in a watertight manner. Janzen and associates[25] from the University of California-Los Angeles (UCLA) evaluated in a porcine model, the safety and efficacy of cryoablation and RFA of cortical and deep renal tissue. Hematoxylin and eosin staining on acute (2 hours) cryolesions demonstrated uniform coagulative necrosis of renal parenchyma and chronic (30 days) cryolesions demonstrated uniform necrosis with fibrous scar formation. Interlobar artery (adjacent to renal pyramid) preservation occurred in seven of 13 (54%) acute and five of nine (56%) chronic cryolesions. Urothelial architecture was preserved in eight of 13 (62%) acute and seven of nine (78%) chronic cryolesions. Hematoxylin and eosin staining on acute and chronic RFA lesions demonstrated indeterminate necrosis, although triphenyl tetrazolium chloride staining of gross specimens confirmed necrosis most definitively in renal cortex. Interlobar artery preservation occurred in six of 13 (46%) acute and three of four (75%) chronic RFA lesions. Urothelial architecture was preserved in one of 13 (8%) acute and two of four (50%) chronic RFA lesions. Acute cryolesion dimensions measured by laparoscopic ultrasound equaled or underestimated lesion size measured grossly in all six cases. Lesion dimensions measured by transcutaneous ultrasound equaled or underestimated true lesion size in three of six cases. In three of six lesions transcutaneous ultrasound overestimated true lesion size by 20%, 76%, and 260%, respectively. The authors concluded that renal cortical tissue can be effectively destroyed by cryoablation or RFA, but treatment of deep parenchymal lesions with either modality may result in incomplete ablation. Furthermore, only cryoablation spared the collecting system, although healing or regress of the urothelium may occur with time after RFA. In addition, laparoscopic ultrasound was more accurate for iceball monitoring than transcutaneous ultrasound. Brashears and associates[27] corroborated these findings by deliberately targeting vital renal structures with cryoablation or RFA. All pigs tolerated the treatment and no procedure-related deaths occurred. Despite significant intentional injury to the collecting system no urinary fistulas were demonstrated in cryoablative specimens (0 of 15). In contrast, damage to the renal pelvis (4 of 7) by dry (3 of 4) or wet (1 of 3) RFA was associated with a high likelihood of urinary extravasation.

Warlick and colleagues[30] recently reported the sequelae of known radiographic iceball extension into the collecting system in eight patients during percutaneous renal tumor cryoablation. All tumors extended to within 9 mm of the collecting system and one to five cryoprobes were used. The radiographic iceball extended into the collecting system in six patients, and within 3 and 5 mm in the other two. None of the patients developed signs, symptoms, or radiographic evidence of urinary leak, fistula, or obstruction with a minimum follow-up of at least 1 month. This is in support of the existing animal data discussed above and may represent an advantage over RFA for the treatment of central tumors. In humans, some of the cryoablated areas, especially in exophytic lesions, will autoamputate a few months after cryoablation.

RENAL CRYOABLATION EQUIPMENT

Various clinically relevant cryogens are available, the boiling point of each determining the nadir temperature that the specific cryoprobe can produce. The size and efficiency of an iceball are influenced by the physical characteristics of the cryoprobe, such as the nadir temperature and diameter. The cryoprobe is the device used to deliver the freezing temperatures necessary for tissue destruction. It is a vacuum-insulated instrument that becomes cool when circulated with a cryogen such as liquid nitrogen (−195°C). The transition from systems circulating liquid nitrogen to gas-driven probes using the Joule-Thompson principle in which pressurized gas is permitted to depressurize through a narrow nozzle located at the tip of the probe, permits the use of ultra-thin probes. In accordance with the gas coefficient and the dimension of the nozzle, different gaseous elements generate different thermal exchange events at the area close to the nozzle. Argon gas is used for cooling (−185.7°C), and helium is used for heating (67°C) the surrounding tissue.

Cryoprobes are available in a variety of models and diameters (1.5–8 mm) suitable for open, laparoscopic, and percutaneous use. Larger probes are capable of creating larger lesions. However, one potential area of concern revolves around the use of the standard, larger cryoprobes of 3–8 mm, noted to cause renal capsular and parenchymal fractures, which can result in significant bleeding.[31] At UCLA, multiple ultrathin 17-gauge (1.47 mm), third-generation cryoprobes (Oncura, Plymouth Meeting, PA, USA) have been used simultaneously for selected patients with small renal tumors.[32] This approach is based on an iceball geometry in which a 9-mm radius is achieved at 5 minutes of continuous freezing, and a 13-mm radius is achieved at 10 minutes of continuous freezing, with the lethal −20°C isotherm located at a radius of 7 mm and 10 mm, respectively. The leading edge of the iceball that is seen on ultrasound, which achieves a freezing temperature of only 0°C, is just 2–3 mm beyond the −20°C zone, allowing a comfortable margin of error if one freezes 5–10 mm beyond the tumor margin on ultrasound. Spacing the probes at 10-mm intervals generates one large iceball created by the confluence of individual, overlapping iceballs.

INDICATIONS AND CONTRAINDICATIONS

Cryoablation should be reserved for select patients with a small renal tumor in order to achieve the goal of reliable complete cancer cell kill. The indications and limitations of this technology are still evolving. The current indications for laparoscopic-assisted renal cryoablation at the authors' institution include small (<3 cm) solitary renal tumors located away from the collecting system in an elderly patient. For posterior tumors <2 cm, percutaneous renal cryoablation can be considered. Open renal cryoablation can be considered in centrally located tumors in a solitary kidney that may pose a challenge to surgical extirpation or in patients with multiple renal tumors due to a hereditary renal cancer syndrome. For larger (>3 cm) tumors, a significantly larger iceball is necessary, requiring the use of more cryoprobes, which increases not only the technical complexity of the procedure but also the potential for inadequate cryoablation, leaving residual viable cancer cells. Given the current lack of 5-year follow-up data, renal cryoablation remains developmental, and the patient must be so cautioned. Contraindications for laparoscopic-assisted renal cryoablation include coagulopathy, significant post-surgical adhesions, and a completely intrarenal, centrally located tumor abutting the renal sinus or hilum. In addition, younger patients should also be excluded.

ADVANTAGES

Renal cryoablation has potential advantages over partial nephrectomy such as decreased blood loss, no renal hilar clamping or warm ischemia, a low complication rate, rapid recovery, and minimal morbidity.[33] Complete obliteration of the renal tumor, including a surrounding margin of healthy kidney tissue, can be confidently performed under ultrasound guidance. There appears to be little question that cryoablation reliably kills kidney cancer cells if performed in a technically competent manner. Intraoperative ultrasound monitoring of the evolving cryolesion is precise, reliable, and reproducible. During follow-up, the lack of a continued decrease in cryolesion size or persistent suspicious radiologic findings must be thoroughly investigated, and may require additional treatment.[31,33–35]

RENAL CRYOABLATION TECHNIQUES

Open

The authors have recently published their technique for open renal cryosurgery in a patient with von Hippel–Lindau disease, and a multisegment, internet-based video tutorial of this surgical technique can be viewed at http://www.elsevier.com/locate/urologyonline.[32] With the patient in a flank position, the kidney is exposed using an extraperitoneal, extrapleural approach. An intraoperative frozen needle biopsy of the lesion is obtained. Real-time B-mode ultrasonography using a 7.5-MHz linear array probe is used with color-flow Doppler to assess tumor size, depth of the parenchymal lesion, and the mass relationship to the collecting system and major vessels. Multiple cryoprobes (17-gauge) are placed at 1-cm intervals along the periphery, base, and center of the tumor in order to form a wedge-shaped lesion. Tip positioning is guided by ultrasound. Cryoablation is initiated by producing tip temperatures reaching −180°C. Freezing continues until the iceball is advanced 10 mm beyond the tumor edge. Ultrasound is used to confirm normal blood flow to the surrounding kidney and obliteration of flow to the ablated lesion. Following a second freeze–thaw cycle, the probe tracts are inspected to ensure hemostasis.

Laparoscopic

The essential technical requirements of renal cryoablation are the same regardless of how it is performed. The procedure involves real-time imaging of the tumor; preplanning of the precise angle and depth of cryoprobe entry; needle biopsy of the tumor for histologic tissue diagnosis; insertion of the cryoprobe perpendicularly through the center of the tumor and advancement up to, or just beyond, the inner (deep) margin of the tumor, ensuring that the active cryoprobe or iceball are not in physical proximity to any adjacent viscera or structure; creation of an iceball approximately 1 cm larger than the size of the tumor to completely engulf the tumor under real-time radiologic monitoring; and the achievement of renal hemostasis following cryoablation. The laparoscopic technique resembles the open approach, but uses instruments modified for laparoscopy, including an intraoperative, laparoscopic ultrasound probe.[36,37] The choice between a transperitoneal and retroperitoneal approach is dictated by the location of the lesion and surgeon preference. The retroperitoneal approach offers the advantage of a decreased risk of bowel injury and the formation of adhesions. However, blunt dissection in this approach is associated with an increased risk for bleeding.[32] An advantage of the laparoscopic approach over the percutaneous approach is that it permits the dual control of direct laparoscopic visualization and ultrasonographic monitoring to ensure the creation of an adequate iceball.[34]

Percutaneous

The percutaneous approach uses the Seldinger technique to position sheaths in the kidney under ultrasound, CT, or MRI guidance in the vicinity of renal lesions. Cryoprobes are then placed through these sheaths and cryoablation is initiated. Uchida and colleagues[19] were the first to report the clinical application of cryoablation to RCC using a percutaneous technique with ultrasound guidance. The development of small-diameter cryoprobes has allowed for the direct placement through a template without making incisions or using tract dilatation and insertion kits.[38] Technical difficulties in monitoring the size of the iceball have been reported.[39]

Monitoring

Intracorporeal ultrasonography is used for both laparoscopic and open approaches, whereas open MRI is used for percutaneous cryoablation. Ultrasound can detect renal tumors, reliably guide a cryoprobe to the target lesion, and capture the characteristic change in appearance of cryoablated tissue. The cryolesion appears as a hypoechoic area with a hyperechoic rim that expands as the freezing process goes on. At the time of thawing, the hyperechoic rim disappears. Animal studies have shown excellent correlation between the ultrasonographic image of the lesion and its diameter measured by calipers.[24,40] Contact ultrasonography with a laparoscopic flexible color Doppler probe is accurate in measuring the size of the evolving renal cryolesion, with a correlation quotient of 0.9295 ($P = 0.0001$).[19]

SURVEILLANCE FOLLOWING RENAL CRYOABLATION

Follow-up protocol following renal cryoablation involves stringent radiologic, histologic, and renal functional evaluation. The Cleveland Clinic recommends that serial MRI with and without gadolinium enhancement be performed on postoperative day 1 and at 1, 3, 6, 12, 18, and 24 months. Thereafter, annual MRI scanning is recommended for 5 years. The maximal diameter of each cryolesion is measured on each sequential MRI scan. At 6 months postoperatively, CT-directed core needle biopsy of the cryoablated tumor is performed for histopathologic examination. Chest radiography and serum creatinine measurements are recommended on a semiannual or annual basis. At UCLA, CT of the abdomen and pelvis with intravenous contrast is performed at 3-month intervals and routine postoperative biopsy of cryolesions is not performed unless the lesion demonstrates residual enhancement.

RESULTS: ONCOLOGIC EFFICACY

Renal cryoablation has been performed by open,[41,42] laparoscopic,[22,31,33,34,36,43] and percutaneous[19,44–46] techniques (Table 9.1). Immediate postoperative and intermediate-term efficacy has been assessed by the radiographic appearance of lesions at various intervals. Rukstalis and colleagues[42] define their radiographic response criteria as initial evidence of infarction and hemorrhage, subsequent obliteration or reduction in size of the renal mass, and absence of growth on radiologic follow-up examinations. They reported on one patient with an enhancing mass unchanged in size at 3 months following surgery. Biopsy showed a microscopic focus of grade 1 RCC and a repeat cryosurgery was eventually performed with a good local control. Atypical enhancement

Table 9. 1 Selective renal cryoablation clinical series

Series	No. of patients	Average lesion size (cm)	Length of follow-up (months)	Percent coming to nephrectomy	No. developing metastasis
Open					
Rukstalis et al 2001[42]	29	2.2[†] (1–4.7)	16 (1–43)	0	0
Laparoscopic					
Rodriguez et al 2000[56]	7*	2.2	14.2	0	0
Lee et al 2003[62]	20	2.6 (1.4–4.5)	14.2 (1–40)	0	0
Nadler et al 2003[43]	15	2.2 (1.2–3.2)	15.1 (5–27)	13.3	0
Cestari et al 2004[31]	37	2.6 (1–6)	20.5 (1–36)	2.8	0
Gore et al 2005[34]	4	2 (1.5–2.5)	8–17	0	0
Gill et al 2005[33]	56	2.3 (1–5)	36	3.6	0
Percutaneous					
Uchida et al 1995[19]	2	Not stated	10	0	2
Shingleton & Sewell, 2004[46]	90	3	30	0	0
Gupta et al 2005[63]	12	2.5	8	0	0
Silverman et al 2005[38]	23	2.6	14 (4–30)	0	0

† Median size.
* Includes laparoscopic and open approach.

on CT or MRI should not be considered a failure unless associated with persistence or growth of the mass. Ankem and associates[35] evaluated the MRI appearance of renal masses (range 1.5–3.5 cm, mean 2.25 cm) in 17 patients following laparoscopic cryoablation. On the first follow-up MRI, five of 17 lesions demonstrated an increase in size and of these five lesions, three had subsequent decrease in size compared to the preoperative size. One patient had peripheral rim enhancement at the previously cryoablated site with nodular enhancement in the subsequent follow-up scans and biopsy was consistent with persistent RCC. This patient underwent partial nephrectomy. The other patient had no further nodular enhancement with decrease in size of the cryoablated site. These authors concluded that enhancement is a clearer indication of recurrence, and that rim enhancement with an increase in size is more concerning than rim enhancement immediately postoperative.

Harmon and associates[47] recently reported a 5% rate of persistent cancer and 2.5% chance of metachronous lesions in a multicenter review of 120 patients who underwent renal cryoablation. Failure was identified at a median of 14 months with a median of three MRIs. All persistent cancers demonstrated enhancement with gadolinium and an increase in size predicted failure in 100% of cases. Median preoperative lesion size of failures was 4 cm (range 3–6 cm). Seventy percent of failures were clear cell RCC, Fuhrman grade I or II, and 10% grade IV. These authors concluded that risk factors for failure following renal cryoablation included size >4 cm and radiographic evidence of growth. Furthermore, radiographic long-term follow-up with MRI or CT was required because failure could be identified more than 14 months from treatment.

Rukstalis and colleagues[42] evaluated the safety and efficacy of open renal cryoablation of small solid renal masses in 29 patients. The median preoperative lesion size
was 2.2 cm, with 22 solid renal masses and seven complex renal lesions. Five serious
adverse events occurred in five patients, with only one event directly related to the
procedure. One patient experienced a biopsy-proven local recurrence, and 91.3%
of patients (median follow-up 16 months) demonstrated a complete radiographic
response with only a residual scar or small, non-enhancing cyst. These authors concluded that open renal cryoablation appeared to be a safe technique for the *in situ*
destruction of solid or complex renal masses and that inadequate freezing may
result in local disease persistence.

Two series, one laparoscopic and one percutaneous, have reported the largest clinical experiences to date. The laparoscopic technique offers distinct procedural advantages, namely a minimally invasive approach, direct visualization of the tumor,
isolation of the cryoprobe and iceball, thus minimizing the chances of contact injury
to adjacent organs, and dual (laparoscopic and ultrasound) monitoring of the evolving iceball, thus enhancing accuracy. In one of the largest clinical reports to date,
laparoscopic cryoablation was performed in 32 patients with a mean tumor size of
2.3 cm.[22] Using the transperitoneal ($n = 10$) or retroperitoneal ($n = 22$) laparoscopic
approach, a double freeze–thaw cycle was performed. The mean surgical time was
2.9 hours; the cryoablation time was 15.1 minutes; and the blood loss was 66.8 ml.
The mean intraoperative ultrasonographic tumor size was 2 cm and the mean cryolesion size 3.2 cm. The hospital stay was less than 23 hours in 69% of patients.
Sequential MRI demonstrated gradual contraction of cryolesion size.[48] The mean
cryolesion diameters postoperatively at day 1 and at 1, 2, 3, and 6 months were
3.5, 3.2, 2.7, 2.1, and 1.8 cm, representing a size reduction of 8%, 23%, 40%, and 48%,
respectively.[22] In the 20 patients who completed 1-year follow-up, no cryolesion
could be identified on MRI scanning in five patients, and a mean size reduction in
the cryolesion of 66% was noted in the remaining 15 patients. Lin and associates[49]
from the Cleveland Clinic reported the first case of complete documentation of total
cancer ablation in a previously cryoablated human renal tumor in a 61-year-old
patient with metachronous bilateral renal cell carcinoma treated with open partial
nephrectomy and subsequently laparoscopic cryoablation. The patient's renal function deteriorated, prompting bilateral radical nephrectomy prior to renal transplantation. Detailed histopathologic examination of the specimen did not reveal any
evidence of malignancy in two cryoablated sites at 36 months (left kidney) and
19 months (right kidney) after the respective cryoablations.

The laparoscopic cryoablation series by Gill and colleagues[33] has now been updated
to 150 patients. Of these, 56 initial patients have now individually completed a minimal follow-up of 3 years each. In these 56 patients, the mean age was 65.2 years
(range 28–84). The mean tumor size was 2.3 cm, with 80% of tumors less than 3 cm
in size and only two tumors abutting the collecting system. All laparoscopic procedures were completed successfully without open conversion, and no kidney was
lost. The mean cryoablation time was 19.5 minutes and mean blood loss was 87 ml,
blood transfusion was necessary in one patient, and the mean hospital stay was 1.7
days. Major complications occurred in two patients (4%): splenic hematoma managed
conservatively in one and heart failure in one. Intraoperative needle biopsy prior to
cryoablation revealed RCC in 60% of patients and oncocytoma in 10%. For a mean
tumor size of 2.3 cm, the mean intraoperative size of the created cryolesion was 3.6 cm.
Serial postoperative MRI scans revealed gradual contraction of the cryoablated

tumor over time: at 1 day, 3 months, 6 months, and 1, 2, and 3 years, the mean cryo-lesion size was 3.7, 2.8, 2.3, 1.7, 1.2, and 0.9 cm, respectively. This represented a spontaneous decrease in tumor size by 26%, 39%, 56%, 69%, and 75%, at 3 months, 6 months, and 1, 2, and 3 years, respectively. At 3 years, 38% of tumors were unde-tectable on MRI; 4% were undetectable at 3 months, 8% at 6 months, 18% at 12 months, 32% at 24 months, and 38% at 36 months. The rate of reduction in cryole-sion size was comparable between tumors when stratified according to intraopera-tive precryoablation needle biopsy results (20 benign vs. 36 RCC). At 6 months, postoperative CT-directed percutaneous 18-gauge core needle biopsy (one to five cores per patient; mean two) data were available for 39 patients (70%). One to five needle cores (mean two) were obtained per patient with a spring-loaded, 18-gauge core biopsy device. Of the 78 total needle cores obtained, RCC was identified in two patients; both patients subsequently underwent secondary laparoscopic radical nephrectomy, and have had no radiological evidence of locally recurrent or metasta-tic disease at a follow-up of 2.5 and 3 years. In the remaining patients, 6-month needle biopsy revealed varying evidence of irreversible cell death, including fibrosis in 21 (53%), hemosiderin deposits in 11 (28%), and coagulative necrosis in five (12%).

In the 51 patients undergoing cryoablation in the setting of a sporadic unilateral renal tumor, 3-year cancer-specific survival was 98%.[33] One patient died of metastatic prostate cancer. Four patients died of metastatic disease in the setting of bilateral RCC. These four patients with bilateral RCC had previously undergone contralat-eral radical or partial nephrectomy prior to unilateral cryoablation. Three-year overall patient survival was 89%. Cryoablation had minimal impact on the renal functional status of the entire study group. Preoperative serum creatinine was 1.2 mg/dl and postoperative serum creatinine was 1.4 mg/dl. New, *de novo* lesions, remote from the cryoablated site, developed in three patients (5.4%). In 10 patients undergoing cryoablation for tumor in a solitary kidney, the mean iceball size was 4.3 cm, mean preoperative serum creatinine was 2.2 mg/dl, and late postoperative serum creatinine was 2.6 mg/dl at a mean follow-up of 43 months. Furthermore, in 13 patients with preexisting baseline renal dysfunction and a mean created iceball size of 4.1 cm mean preoperative and postoperative serum creatinine measurements were similar (3.0 and 2.7 mg/dl, respectively). None of the 56 patients required con-version to open surgery, none developed a urinary fistula or required dialysis, and none developed a perirenal or port site recurrence.[33]

Desai and co-workers[50] have retrospectively compared the intraoperative charac-teristics and intermediate-term follow-up of 78 patients that underwent laparoscopic renal cryoablation to 153 patients that underwent laparoscopic partial nephrectomy for renal tumors ≤3 cm. Patients undergoing laparoscopic partial nephrectomy were younger (mean age, 60.6 vs. 65.6 years; $P = 0.005$), healthier (American Society of Anesthesiologists class 3/4 present in 46% vs. 75%; $P = 0.001$), had a lower baseline serum creatinine (90.1 vs. 106.0 µmol/L [1.02 vs. 1.2 mg/dl]; $P = 0.01$), a larger tumor size (2.3 vs. 2.1 cm; $P = 0.02$), and fewer cases of solitary kidneys (5% vs. 23%; $P = 0.000$). Laparoscopic partial nephrectomy was associated with greater blood loss (211 vs. 101 ml; $P = 0.000$) and a higher incidence of delayed complications after hospital discharge (16.3% vs. 2.2%; $P = 0.01$) compared with cryoablation. Both groups were comparable with regard to operative time, intraoperative complica-tions, postoperative complications, hospital stay, convalescence, and postoperative serum creatinine (112.2 vs. 123.7 µmol/L [1.27 vs 1.4 mg/dl]; $P = 0.31$). There were two local recurrences (3%) in the laparoscopic renal cryoablation group detected over a mean follow-up of 24.6 months and one local recurrence (0.6%) in the laparo-scopic partial nephrectomy group detected over a mean follow-up time of 5.8 months. Laparoscopic renal cryoablation was technically simpler to perform and was associated with a lower incidence of major complications and blood loss compared to laparoscopic partial nephrectomy.

Percutaneous cryoablation with open-magnet MRI monitoring in 20 patients was reported by Shingleton and Sewell.[44] The mean tumor size was 3 cm, operative time was 1.5 hours, and hospital stay was 23 hours for 95% of the patients. In a more recent update with 90 patients with enhancing renal masses less than 5 cm in size treated by MRI-guided cryoablation, these investigators reported that 92% of patients had successful tumor ablation at median follow-up of 30 months. Follow-up MRIs were obtained at 1, 3, and every 6 months thereafter. There were nine complications, one major (perinephric hemorrhage) and eight minor (one UTI, one wound infection, five flank paresthesia, one respiratory difficulty). Postoperative histologic and/or long-term sequential radiologic data with measurements of individual cryolesion size were not reported for the entire study group. Silverman and associates[38] recently evaluated 26 renal tumors (diameter range, 1.0–4.6 cm; mean, 2.6 cm) in 23 patients that were treated with 27 MRI-guided percutaneous cryoablation procedures. Of 26 masses, 24 were RCC, one was a transitional cell carcinoma, and one was an angiomyolipoma. Tumors were considered successfully ablated if they demon-strated no contrast enhancement at follow-up CT or MR imaging (mean, 14 months; range, 4–30 months). Twenty-four of 26 (93%) tumors were successfully ablated, 23 of which required only one treatment session. Two complications occurred in a total of 27 cryoablations: one hemorrhage, which required a blood transfusion, and one abscess, which was treated successfully with percutaneous catheter drainage.

In the series by Shingleton and Sewell,[44] the renal lesions were treated without performing a pretreatment biopsy. In a recent report by Frank and co-workers,[51] 46% of renal masses of less than 1 cm were determined to be benign after surgical resection. A smaller lesion is considered a favorable characteristic for percutaneous ablative therapy; therefore, a significant fraction of patients undergoing percutaneous ablative therapy can be expected to have benign lesions. This should be kept in mind when evaluating outcomes and the oncologic efficacy of the treatment should not be overstated. Ideally, when evaluating a new therapy, outcomes such as recurrence rates and survival should be evaluated only in patients with biopsy-proven cancer, and patients with benign disease should be excluded.

COMPLICATIONS

No worsening of renal function following renal cryoablation has been reported. Hemorrhage, thrombosis, and urinary fistula formation are all potential risks of cryoablation; however, few if any of these complications have been noted. Table 9.2 shows reported complications of renal cryoablation in selective clinical studies. Complications of cryoablation noted in animal models, but not in humans, include freezing of the collecting system in a dog without evidence of urinary leakage or hemorrhage,[28] and secondary ureteropelvic junction stricture.[21] Cracking and bleeding of renal parenchyma during the thaw phase have been noted by some groups during open as well as laparoscopic cryoablation.[52] Electrocautery, surgical mesh, avitene plugs, thrombin-soaked gel foam, cellulose mesh, and argon beam laser application have all been used to establish hemostasis in laparoscopic procedures when cracking

Table 9.2 Frequency of complications of cryoablation in selective clinical studies*

	Urinary extravasation	Postop hemorrhage	Renal capsule fracture	Renal failure requiring dialysis	Liver laceration	Postop CHF	Pelvic vein thrombosis
Open							
Delworth et al 1996[41]	0/2	0/2	0/2	0/2	0/2	0/2	0/2
Zegel et al 1998[64]	0/6	0/6	0/6	0/6	0/6	0/6	0/6
Rukstalis et al 2001[42]	0/29	0/29	4/29	3/29	0/29	1/29	0/29
Laparoscopic							
Bishoff et al 1999[65]	0/9	0/9	0/9	0/9	0/9	0/9	0/9
Gill et al 2000[22]	0/32	0/32	0/32	0/32	1/32	0/32	0/32
Rodriguez et al 2000[56]	0/7	0/7	0/7	0/7	0/7	0/7	1/7
Cestari et al 2004[31]	0/37	2/37	3/37	0/37	0/37	0/37	0/37
Gill et al 2005[33]	0/56	0/56	0/56	0/56	†1/56	1/56	0/56
Percutaneous							
Uchida et al 1995[19]	0/2	0/2	0/2	0/2	0/2	0/2	0/2
Silverman et al 2005[38]	0/27	1/27	0/27	0/27	0/27	0/27	0/27

Postop, postoperative; CHF, congestive heart failure.
†Splenic hematoma.
*Values are expressed as frequency/n.

and bleeding have occurred. At UCLA, fibrin glue is inserted into the probe tract while still frozen in order to prevent bleeding following thawing.

Renal cryoablation does not lead to any clinically significant systemic hypothermia. The ischemic necrotic renal cryolesion, which remains *in situ*, does not seem to trigger renin–angiotensin-mediated hypertension or have a deleterious impact on renal function over a long-term follow-up of up to 20 months.[53] Renal cryoablation does not adversely alter urinary composition with respect to lithogenic parameters for up to 2 months after surgery. Elevated urinary beta-2 microglobulin levels indicating significant renal injury immediately following cryoabation spontaneously revert to baseline levels within 2 months.[54]

Johnson and colleagues[55] recently identified in a multi-institutional review, complications that were associated with percutaneous and laparoscopic ablative treatment for renal tumors. Mean experience at each individual institution was 68 cases (range 21–92). A total of 30 complications occurred (11.1%) with five major (1.8% or two in the cryoablation and three in the RFA group) and 25 minor (9.2% or 17 in the cryoablation and eight in the RFA group) complications, and one death (0.4%) in the RFA group. A total of 20 complications (14.4%) occurred after cryoablation (four after laparoscopic and 16 after percutaneous ablation) and 10 (7.6%) occurred after RFA (six after percutaneous and four after laparoscopic ablation). The reported death occurred 3 days after percutaneous RFA. The complication rate decreased with experience, with 16 (53.3%), five (16.6%) and nine (30.0%) of the 30 complications occurring in the initial, intermediate, and latest third of the case experiences, respectively. All five major complications occurred in the initial third of patients in each center experience. The death occurred in the final third of patients. The most common complication was pain or paresthesia at the percutaneous probe insertion site. This accounted for 46.6% of all complications (14 of 30) and occurred in 5.2% of all cases (14 of 271). Of the 30 complications, 25 (83.3%) were directly attributable to the ablation procedure. Two of the remaining five patients had post-procedure pneumonia. A third patient had respiratory difficulty after the procedure with a negative pulmonary angiogram and no clear cause of the problem. The other two patients were diagnosed with a urinary tract infection after ablative treatment. The five major complications included one case of open conversion due to inability to access the tumor laparoscopically, one case of ileus after laparoscopic RFA that required hospital readmission, one episode of hemorrhage after percutaneous cryoablation that required reoperation for control, self-limited and subclinical urine leakage through the ablated needle tract seen only on retrograde pyelogram and one case of ureteropelvic junction (UPJ) obstruction caused by scarring secondary to RFA tissue damage. Of these patients the first four recovered fully and the UPJ obstruction led to loss of renal function and eventual nephrectomy. The single death was attributed to post-procedure aspiration pneumonia in a patient with poor overall health, including a history of chronic obstructive pulmonary disease, congestive heart failure, and pulmonary histoplasmosis. This death was not considered directly attributable to the ablation technique, but rather to a surgical procedure in a debilitated individual. In the subgroup of 90 laparoscopic procedures, eight complications occurred (8.9%), of which three were attributable to laparoscopic technique (3.3%), four were to the ablation procedure (4.4%) and one was iatrogenic (pneumonia).

Cestari and colleagues[31] reported their experience with laparoscopic renal cryoablation using liquid nitrogen-based ErbeCryo 6 (ErBE Elektromedizin GmBH, Baden-Wuerttemberg, Germany) sharp-tip, reusable 3.2-mm cryoprobes. Postoperative complications included three cases of transitory hyperthermia, hematoma (with previous renal fracture) in the surgical area in two, and gross hematuria in one, of which all were treated conservatively. A delayed complication was UPJ obstruction in one case due to retraction of the cryolesion, which required pyeloplasty 8 months after surgery. Mean follow-up was 20.54 months (range 1–36). These authors state that renal fracture was due to an excessive angle of cryoprobe insertion into the renal mass and was typically associated with increased bleeding at the end of the second thawing phase. They recommended that it was essential to insert the probe into the kidney as perpendicularly as possible, maintain the probe in as fixed a position as possible during the procedure, and remove the probe after the second thawing phase only when the tissue had completely thawed.

LIMITATIONS

Ablative techniques do not generate pathologic specimens that allow accurate pathologic diagnosis and thus preclude accurate tissue diagnosis, staging, and grading, which are important for prognosis determination. Therefore, biopsy of perirenal fat and of the renal mass is promoted by some investigators. However, the reliability of such biopsies has been called into question. Moreover, performing pretreatment biopsy during percutaneous procedures may potentially cause tract seeding. Thus, reliable freezing and complete eradication of tissue with achievement of adequate margins during the procedure needs to be ensured. Debate continues to exist over which of two techniques of intraoperative monitoring is preferable: use of thermocouples, as advocated by Rodriguez and associates[56] or following radiographic lesion appearance, as advocated by Gill and co-workers.[22] Concern for achieving negative margins has led some investigators to modify their techniques in order to obtain pathologic specimens.

A primary critique of renal cryosurgery is the lack of histologic confirmation of the completeness of tumor destruction. Unlike partial nephrectomy, in which the tumor is excised, the *in situ* nature of ablative techniques, such as cryoablation, precludes histologic evaluation of the surgical margins. As such, meticulous and dedicated long-term clinical and radiologic follow-up are necessary to document the oncologic outcomes and to determine the local recurrence and cancer-free survival rates. Although port site tumor seeding during laparoscopic-assisted or percutaneous cryoablation is a theoretical concern, the authors' are unaware of any reported case to date.

FUTURE DIRECTIONS

Various adjunctive cryoenhancers are being investigated to maximize the completeness of cryoinjury, targeted especially at the so-called zone of sublethal destruction located at the periphery of the iceball.[57] Chemotherapeutic agents, such as cyclophosphamide, 5-fluorouracil (5-FU), and bleomycin, administered systemically or injected directly into the tumor just after thawing may have synergistic cytocidal effect by prompting apoptosis due to high local tissue drug levels. A combination of freezing and 5-FU produced more complete cell kill than by either modality alone. Radiotherapy may potentially confer benefits, since freezing enhances the radiosensitivity of cells.[58,59] Direct injection of antifreeze proteins into the tumor may enhance the destructive effects of freezing.[60,61] Lastly, imaging of the evolving cryolesion with electrical impedance tomography may increase the accuracy of real-time monitoring.[57]

CONCLUSIONS

Minimally invasive modalities for the treatment of RCC are being introduced as new nephron-sparing approaches in an attempt to minimize operative time, morbidity, and time to full recovery. Of the probe-ablative techniques currently available for renal tumors, cryoablation is the most studied and clinically applied procedure. The targeted tissue is rapidly frozen *in situ*, followed by sloughing of the devitalized tissue and healing by secondary intention over time. The established essential features of cryoablation include rapid freezing, slow thawing, and repetition of the freeze–thaw cycle. Advantages of cryoablation include predictable clearly necrotic lesions that can be monitored reliably with real-time imaging. Nevertheless, because the ablated tumor is left *in situ*, the lack of histologic data on complete tumor destruction and the adequacy of negative surgical margins remain a central critique. There is ongoing optimization of treatment modalities and refinement of techniques. Long-term studies are needed to confirm a durable response compared to partial and radical nephrectomy. Nevertheless, inclusion criteria based on size, location, and type of treatable lesions and patient selection continue to evolve. Renal cryoablation is generally reserved for exophytic lesions <3 cm. It can also serve older patients with significant comorbidities. The role of percutaneous techniques is still unclear. Radiographic follow-up is essential. The best modality (i.e. MRI, ultrasound, or CT) for tumor targeting, monitoring of therapy, and follow-up is still under investigation. For minimally invasive cryoablative measures to gain a place as nephron-sparing approaches, it should show both equivalent efficacy and reduced morbidity relative to those of open partial nephrectomy. At this time, these techniques must be considered developmental and should be reserved for carefully selected patients and should be compared to the evolving modality of laparoscopic partial nephrectomy.

REFERENCES

1. Lam JS, Shvarts O, Leppert JT et al. Renal cell carcinoma 2005: new frontiers in staging, prognostication and targeted molecular therapy. J Urol 2005; 173: 1853–62.
2. Robson CJ, Churchill BM, Anderson W. The results of radical nephrectomy for renal cell carcinoma. J Urol 1969; 101: 297–301.
3. Bosniak MA. Observation of small incidentally detected renal masses. Semin Urol Oncol 1995; 13: 267–72.
4. Volpe A, Panzarella T, Rendon RA et al. The natural history of incidentally detected small renal masses. Cancer 2004; 100: 738–45.
5. Kassouf W, Aprikian AG, Laplante M, Tanguay S. Natural history of renal masses followed expectantly. J Urol 2004; 171: 111–13; discussion 113.
6. Kato M, Suzuki T, Suzuki Y et al. Natural history of small renal cell carcinoma: evaluation of growth rate, histological grade, cell proliferation and apoptosis. J Urol 2004; 172: 863–6.
7. Smith SJ, Bosniak MA, Megibow AJ et al. Renal cell carcinoma: earlier discovery and increased detection. Radiology 1989; 170: 699–703.
8. Palmer JM. Role of partial nephrectomy in solitary or bilateral renal tumors. JAMA 1983; 249: 2357–61.
9. Novick AC. Partial nephrectomy for renal cell carcinoma. Urol Clin North Am 1987; 14: 419–33.
10. Herr HW. Partial nephrectomy for renal cell carcinoma with a normal opposite kidney. Cancer 1994; 73: 160–2.

11. Belldegrun A, Tsui KH, deKernion JB, Smith RB. Efficacy of nephron-sparing surgery for renal cell carcinoma: analysis based on the new 1997 tumor–node–metastasis staging system. J Clin Oncol 1999; 17: 2868–75.
12. Lau WK, Blute ML, Weaver AL et al. Matched comparison of radical nephrectomy vs nephron-sparing surgery in patients with unilateral renal cell carcinoma and a normal contralateral kidney. Mayo Clin Proc 2000; 75: 1236–42.
13. D'Armiento M, Damiano R, Feleppa B et al. Elective conservative surgery for renal carcinoma versus radical nephrectomy: a prospective study. Br J Urol 1997; 79: 15–19.
14. Lerner SE, Hawkins CA, Blute ML et al. Disease outcome in patients with low stage renal cell carcinoma treated with nephron sparing or radical surgery. J Urol 1996; 155: 1868–73.
15. Lee CT, Katz J, Shi W et al. Surgical management of renal tumors 4 cm or less in a contemporary cohort. J Urol 2000; 163: 730–6.
16. Lam JS, Shvarts O, Leppert JT et al. Postoperative surveillance protocol for patients with localized and locally advanced renal cell carcinoma based on a validated prognostic nomogram and risk group stratification system. J Urol 2005; 174: 466–72.
17. Patard JJ, Shvarts O, Lam JS et al. Safety and efficacy of partial nephrectomy for all T1 tumors based on an international multicenter experience. J Urol 2004; 171: 2181–5, quiz 2435.
18. Leibovich BC, Blute ML, Cheville JC et al. Nephron sparing surgery for appropriately selected renal cell carcinoma between 4 and 7 cm results in outcome similar to radical nephrectomy. J Urol 2004; 171: 1066–70.
19. Uchida M, Imaide Y, Sugimoto K et al. Percutaneous cryosurgery for renal tumours. Br J Urol 1995; 75: 132–6; discussion 136–7.
20. Baust J, Gage AA, Ma H, Zhang CM. Minimally invasive cryosurgery – technological advances. Cryobiology 1997; 34: 373–84.
21. Campbell SC, Krishnamurthi V, Chow G et al. Renal cryosurgery: experimental evaluation of treatment parameters. Urology 1998; 52: 29–33; discussion 33–4.
22. Gill IS, Novick AC, Meraney AM et al. Laparoscopic renal cryoablation in 32 patients. Urology 2000; 56: 748–53.
23. Collyer W, Venkatesh R, Vanlangendonck R et al. Enhanced renal cryoablation with hilar clamping and intrarenal cooling in a porcine model. Urology 2004; 63: 1209–12.
24. Stephenson RA, King DK, Rohr LR. Renal cryoablation in a canine model. Urology 1996; 47: 772–6.
25. Janzen NK, Perry KT, Han KR et al. The effects of intentional cryoablation and radio frequency ablation of renal tissue involving the collecting system in a porcine model. J Urol 2005; 173: 1368–74.
26. Ames CD, Vanlangendonck R, Venkatesh R et al. Enhanced renal parenchymal cryoablation with novel 17-gauge cryoprobes. Urology 2004; 64: 173–5.
27. Brashears JH 3rd, Raj GV, Crisci A et al. Renal cryoablation and radio frequency ablation: an evaluation of worst case scenarios in a porcine model. J Urol 2005; 173: 2160–5.
28. Nakada SY, Lee FT Jr, Warner T et al. Laparoscopic cryosurgery of the kidney in the porcine model: an acute histological study. Urology 1998; 51: 161–6.
29. Sung GT, Gill IS, Hsu TH et al. Effect of intentional cryo-injury to the renal collecting system. J Urol 2003; 170: 619–22.
30. Warlick CA, Lima GC, Allaf ME et al. Collecting system involvement during renal tumor cryoablation. J Urol 2005; 173 (Suppl): 263, abstract 971.
31. Cestari A, Guazzoni G, dell'Acqua V et al. Laparoscopic cryoablation of solid renal masses: intermediate term followup. J Urol 2004; 172: 1267–70.
32. Pantuck AJ, Zisman A, Cohen J, Belldegrun A. Cryosurgical ablation of renal tumors using 1.5-millimeter, ultrathin cryoprobes. Urology 2002; 59: 130–3.
33. Gill IS, Remer EM, Hasan WA et al. Renal cryoablation: outcome at 3 years. J Urol 2005; 173: 1903–7.
34. Gore JL, Kim HL, Schulam P. Initial experience with laparoscopically assisted percutaneous cryotherapy of renal tumors. J Endourol 2005; 19: 480–3.

35. Ankem MK, Moon TD, Hedican SP et al. Is peripheral enhancement a sign of recurrence of renal cell carcinoma post cryoablation? J Urol 2004; 171 (Suppl): 506, abstract 1914.
36. Gill IS, Novick AC, Soble JJ et al. Laparoscopic renal cryoablation: initial clinical series. Urology 1998; 52: 543–51.
37. Johnson DB, Nakada SY. Laparoscopic cryoablation for renal-cell cancer. J Endourol 2000; 14: 873–8; discussion 878–9.
38. Silverman SG, Tuncali K, vanSonnenberg E et al. Renal tumors: MR imaging-guided percutaneous cryotherapy – initial experience in 23 patients. Radiology 2005; 236: 716–24.
39. Long JP, Faller GT. Percutaneous cryoablation of the kidney in a porcine model. Cryobiology 1999; 38: 89–93.
40. Onik GM, Reyes G, Cohen JK, Porterfield B. Ultrasound characteristics of renal cryosurgery. Urology 1993; 42: 212–15.
41. Delworth MG, Pisters LL, Fornage BD, von Eschenbach AC. Cryotherapy for renal cell carcinoma and angiomyolipoma. J Urol 1996; 155: 252–4; discussion 254–5.
42. Rukstalis DB, Khorsandi M, Garcia FU et al. Clinical experience with open renal cryoablation. Urology 2001; 57: 34–9.
43. Nadler RB, Kim SC, Rubenstein JN et al. Laparoscopic renal cryosurgery: the Northwestern experience. J Urol 2003; 170: 1121–5.
44. Shingleton WB, Sewell PE Jr. Percutaneous renal tumor cryoablation with magnetic resonance imaging guidance. J Urol 2001; 165: 773–6.
45. Shingleton WB, Sewell PE Jr. Percutaneous renal cryoablation of renal tumors in patients with von Hippel–Lindau disease. J Urol 2002; 167: 1268–70.
46. Shingleton WB, Sewell PE. Percutaneous renal tumor cryoablation: results in the first 90 patients. J Urol 2004; 171 (Suppl): 463, abstract 1751.
47. Harmon JD, Parulkar BG, Doble A, Rukstalis DB. Critical assessment of cancer recurrence following renal cryoablation: a multi-center review. J Urol 2004; 171 (Suppl): 469, abstract 1775.
48. Remer EM, Weinberg EJ, Oto A et al. MR imaging of the kidneys after laparoscopic cryoablation. AJR Am J Roentgenol 2000; 174: 635–40.
49. Lin CH, Moinzadeh A, Ramani AP, Gill IS. Histopathologic confirmation of complete cancer-cell kill in excised specimens after renal cryotherapy. Urology 2004; 64: 590.
50. Desai MM, Aron M, Gill IS. Laparoscopic partial nephrectomy versus laparoscopic cryoablation for the small renal tumor. Urology 2005; 66: 23–8.
51. Frank I, Blute ML, Cheville JC et al. Solid renal tumors: an analysis of pathological features related to tumor size. J Urol 2003; 170: 2217–20.
52. Cozzi PJ, Lynch WJ, Collins S et al. Renal cryotherapy in a sheep model; a feasibility study. J Urol 1997; 157: 710–12.
53. Carvalhal EF, Gill IS, Meraney AM et al. Laparoscopic renal cryoablation: impact on renal function and blood pressure. Urology 2001; 58: 357–61.
54. Ng CS, Gill IS. Impact of renal cryoablation on urine composition. Urology 2002; 59: 831–4.
55. Johnson DB, Solomon SB, Su LM et al. Defining the complications of cryoablation and radio frequency ablation of small renal tumors: a multi-institutional review. J Urol 2004; 172: 874–7.
56. Rodriguez R, Chan DY, Bishoff JT et al. Renal ablative cryosurgery in selected patients with peripheral renal masses. Urology 2000; 55: 25–30.
57. Baust JG, Gage AA, Clarke D et al. Cryosurgery – a putative approach to molecular-based optimization. Cryobiology 2004; 48: 190–204.
58. Burton SA, Paljug WR, Kalnicki S, Werts ED. Hypothermia-enhanced human tumor cell radiosensitivity. Cryobiology 1997; 35: 70–8.
59. Znati CA, Werts E, Kociban D, Kalnicki S. Variables influencing response of human prostate carcinoma cells to combined radiation and cryotherapy in vitro. Cryobiology 1998; 37: 450–1.
60. Muldrew K, Rewcastle J, Donnelly BJ et al. Flounder antifreeze peptides increase the efficacy of cryosurgery. Cryobiology 2001; 42: 182–9.

61. Pham L, Dahiya R, Rubinsky B. An in vivo study of antifreeze protein adjuvant cryosurgery. Cryobiology 1999; 38: 169–75.
62. Lee DI, McGinnis DE, Feld R, Strup SE. Retroperitoneal laparoscopic cryoablation of small renal tumors: intermediate results. Urology 2003; 61: 83–8.
63. Gupta A, Allaf ME, Warlick CA et al. Percutaneous renal tumor cryoablation under CT guidance: initial clinical experience. J Urol 2005; 173 (Suppl): 413, abstract 1526.
64. Zegel HG, Holland GA, Jennings SB et al. Intraoperative ultrasonographically guided cryoablation of renal masses: initial experience. J Ultrasound Med 1998; 17: 571–6.
65. Bishoff JT, Chen RB, Lee BR et al. Laparoscopic renal cryoablation: acute and long-term clinical, radiographic, and pathologic effects in an animal model and application in a clinical trial. J Endourol 1999; 13: 233–9.

10

Percutaneous renal cryoablation: state of the art

Leslie A. Deane, Ralph V. Clayman

History of cryotherapy in urology • Experimental evidence for efficacy of tissue cryoablation • Cryobiology and mechanisms of effect • Selection criteria for percutaneous renal cryoablation • Percutaneous renal cryoablation: clinical experience • Technique of percutaneous renal cryoablation using magnetic resonance imaging guidance • Technique of percutaneous renal cryoablation using real-time ultrasound guidance • Technique of percutaneous renal cryoablation using real-time CT fluoroscopic guidance • Post-treatment follow-up: imaging characteristics • Complications of percutaneous renal cryotherapy • Devices and probes currently in clinical use • Future directions

HISTORY OF CRYOTHERAPY IN UROLOGY

Cryotherapy refers to the destruction of tissue by controlled freezing. It was first employed in the 19th century, when advanced malignancies of the breast and cervix were treated with the application of ice-cold saline solution.[1] More recently, it has been applied topically for the treatment of skin cancers using liquid nitrogen and also percutaneously or at open surgery to treat liver and uterine tumors using specially designed cryoprobes. In urological practice, cryotherapy was first used almost 40 years ago to treat benign prostatic hyperplasia;[2] in the 1970s cryotherapy was initially employed in the treatment of prostate cancer, both as primary therapy and for post-radiation recurrent disease.[3] In the last decade the treatment of small renal tumors has become an evolving indication for cryotherapy.

This chapter will focus on the delivery of cryosurgical energy via the percutaneous approach, the technique, results, complications, and follow-up. In addition, the basics of the cryobiology of cryosurgical injury will be highlighted.

EXPERIMENTAL EVIDENCE FOR EFFICACY OF TISSUE CRYOABLATION

In 1992, Long and Faller examined the application of cryosurgical energy to the normal porcine kidney.[4] This was done percutaneously in 13 juvenile swine. The cryogen or the cryoprobe used in this study was not stated. This group employed ultrasound guidance for probe placement. Animals were treated for either 3–4 minutes or 6–7 minutes with a single cryoprobe or for 10 minutes with two parallel probes 2 mm apart. Upon nephrectomy, which was typically between 0 and 42 days post treatment in order to establish a timeline for the histological changes within each group, examination of the kidneys revealed cryolesions of 1–2 cm and 3–4 cm in the kidneys treated for 3–4 minutes and 6–7 minutes, respectively, and there was little perirenal reaction. In the longest treatment group, the cryolesions were 6–7 cm and significant perirenal reaction with engulfing of the ureter and hydronephrosis in two of six kidneys was noted. These latter two kidneys were harvested at 21 and 33 days respectively. There was also adherence to the colon and posterior abdominal wall musculature seen in five of the six kidneys removed between 7 and 33 days post treatment in this longer treatment group. Histologically, lesions were similar in all groups and characterized by confluent areas of central coagulative necrosis with discrete borders. The zone between normal and necrotic regions was no greater than 1–2 mm and characterized by atrophic or metaplastic epithelial remnants. Over time the lesions developed into contracted areas of fibrosis with normal surrounding parenchyma. The size of these areas differed widely, likely due to different post-treatment sacrifice times (0–42 days).

Onik and colleagues,[5] using ultrasound at open laparotomy in five dogs, were able to monitor the progression of the renal cryolesion and correlated its sonographic size with the size at gross examination. They also found coagulative necrosis on histology with a sharp zone of transition from necrotic treated tissue to normal tissue.

Nakada et al[6] in 2000, implanted the kidneys of 80 rabbits with VX2 tumor, in a subcapsular location, in an *in vivo* model of renal cancer. Ten animals were then used as controls and 70 were randomized to cryoablation versus nephrectomy 7 days following implantation. The cryoablation was performed using a double freeze technique delivered through 2.4-mm probes and the argon-based Cryocare System (Endocare, Irvine, CA) with margins targeted to $-20°C$. Animals were harvested at 22 days. Controls uniformly demonstrated metastasis versus metastasis in only 34% and 36% of cryoablated and nephrectomized animals, respectively. The cure rates were therefore similar for cryoablation and for nephrectomy despite this aggressive tumor model.

Shingleton et al[7] treated five kidneys percutaneously in a porcine model with magnetic resonance imaging guidance to create six cryolesions percutaneously. A 3-mm Oncura (Plymouth Meeting, PA) MRI-compatible cryoprobe was used to deliver argon gas at a pressure of 4000 psi and iceball temperature of $-80°C$. The freeze times ranged from 2 to 8 minutes and all animals were sacrificed at 1 week. They identified four zones of injury including a central area of complete coagulative necrosis, a 1-mm thick area of neutrophilic infiltrate, an area of hemorrhage and a surrounding area of regeneration and fibrosis. The size of the cryolesion on imaging correlated with the size at pathological examination.

Employing a laparoscopic technique, Wooley et al[8] treated the normal kidney in 16 female mongrel dogs with single versus double freeze–thaw cycles and active versus passive thaw using the argon gas based Cryocare Cryo surgical system by Endocare (Irvine, CA). A 3-mm cryoprobe by Endocare was used. They found a central area of complete liquefactive necrosis surrounded by granulation and fibrous tissue when the animals were sacrificed at 4 weeks. Interstitial cryoprobe temperatures decreased from 31.3°C to $-142°C$.

In 2003, Sung et al[9] examined the effect of intentionally injuring the collecting system with cryosurgical energy in 12 swine using an open technique. Two groups with a 3-cm versus 4.5-cm iceball were compared. Real-time confirmation of the involvement of the collecting system was demonstrated by retrograde ureteropyelography. Despite complete sloughing of the urothelium, regeneration occurred with increased fibrosis noted in the lamina propria of animals treated with the larger cryolesion versus minimal fibrosis with the smaller cryolesion. These findings were noted when animals were sacrificed at 1 and 3 months. The degree of injury and fibrosis were no different when the renal pelvis was irrigated with warm saline at 38–42°C at 10 ml/min. This study showed that in the absence of direct puncture the collecting system heals by secondary intention and appears relatively immune to cryoablation. However, no mention was made regarding the occurrence of infundibular stenosis.

Rehman et al[10] treated the normal kidney in seven domestic pigs via a laparoscopic approach using argon gas as the cryogen. Seventeen-gauge cryoprobes (Oncura, Plymouth Meeting, PA) were employed and nadir temperatures at the probe tip of −140 to −160°C were recorded. Gross examination demonstrated a thickened and wrinkled capsule which was adherent to the underlying renal parenchyma. Each lesion showed a wedged-shaped area of coagulative necrosis in the cortex and medulla extending to the renal pelvis, with a complete lack of cellular details for all kidney substructures extending from the renal capsule to the collecting system. The urothelium appeared relatively resistant to injury. They also confirmed the ability to monitor the cryolesion sonographically. Lesion size increased when using three probes versus one probe. Of note, the necrosis within the cryolesions was complete; there were no skip areas of viable tissue.

Finally Brashears et al[11] recently evaluated the worst-case scenarios of renal cryoablation (CA) and radiofrequency ablation (RFA) in a porcine model. They deliberately placed the cryoprobe or radiofrequency probe into the renal pelvis (5 CA, 7 RFA), major calyx (5 CA, 5 RFA) or segmental renal vessel (5 CA, 7 RFA) of the animals. Three-centimeter lesions were created by each modality and the kidneys were examined at 10 days by gross sectioning and histologically and also by *ex vivo* retrograde pyelogram. There were no urinary fistulae in the cryoablation group versus four of seven when the renal pelvis was treated in the radiofrequency ablated specimens. Janzen et al[12] also confirmed the absence of collecting system damage in a pig model in which deep parenchymal lesions were treated with cryoablation versus those treated with radiofrequency ablation.

CRYOBIOLOGY AND MECHANISMS OF EFFECT

Several theories have been advanced regarding the mechanism of tissue injury in response to cryosurgery. These include direct cellular injury, vascular injury, and immunologic enhancement. However, the last seems to play a less consistent role.

Direct cellular injury

Two responses of tissue water have been identified and linked to cell injury during freezing. It has been shown that as tissue is cooled, extracellular freezing occurs and results in an increase in the solute concentration in this compartment. This leads to osmotic cellular dehydration, damage to the enzymatic machinery and destabilization of the cell membrane. Secondly, the formation of intracellular ice, occurring when cooling is rapid enough to trap water in the cell, likely damages intracellular organelles and membranes. Thus, at lower cooling rates injury occurs by solute effects and cellular dehydration, whereas at higher rates of cooling damage occurs following intracellular ice formation as water is trapped within the cell and does not have time to equilibrate with the extracellular space.[13,14]

Vascular injury

Injury to the vessel wall appears to be an important factor in the vascular-mediated response to cryotherapy. There are three proposed pathways of vessel wall damage: (a) mechanical injury of the vessel wall due to vessel distention and engorgement from perivascular cellular dehydration; (b) direct injury to the cells lining the vessel; and (c) reperfusion injury to the endothelium. These events led to activation of the coagulation cascade, platelet aggregation, and subsequent thrombosis.[13,14]

Important in the mechanisms cited above is the thermal history of the injury. This refers to the time taken to achieve the target temperature (cooling rate), the minimum temperature (end temperature), the time held at that minimum temperature (hold time), and the thawing rate.

Baust and Gage[15] state that the advancing edge of the iceball as seen on ultrasound as a hyperechoic border is about 0°C. The inner edge of the rim is located 3–4 mm inside of the leading edge or approximately 80% of the distance from the source to the edge of the iceball and is typically in the −20°C isotherm. This group advocates cooling to −40°C to ensure complete tumor kill and notes that this temperature isotherm occurs approximately 60% of the distance from the probe to the ice boundary and 8 mm inside the leading edge of the iceball. Cell kill will, however, be highly dependent on the tissue being treated.

Chosy et al[16] investigated the predictors of renal tissue necrosis in swine treated with a nitrogen-based cryosurgical system. They found that a temperature of −19.4°C or lower was required to ensure complete and homogeneous necrosis. This typically occurred within 16 mm of the 3.4-mm cryoprobes used in this system and was measured by placement of tissue thermocouples. The freeze cycle used was 15 minutes and the minimum temperature at the probe tip was −196°C.

Gage[13] also recommends a slow thaw rate, citing the fact that slower rates produce greater cell damage due to solute effects and maximal growth of ice crystals. These large crystals have an abrasive effect, producing mechanical disruption of cells. Repeating the cycle allows cells to undergo the deleterious physicochemical changes again and with each successive cycle the border of certain destruction is moved closer to the periphery of the frozen volume. Woolley et al[8] also recommend a double freeze–thaw cycle for these reasons.

The optimum duration of freezing is not known. If temperatures are less than −50°C, duration is likely unimportant. However, if the temperature is above −40°C, holding will increase tissue destruction again via solute effects and recrystallization.[13] Most groups have therefore held temperatures for approximately 10–15 minutes.

Immunologic enhancement

Hedican et al[17] presented data on cryotherapy and immune function obtained from a murine renal cell carcinoma model (Renca). Subcapsular implantation of the Renca cell line in 28 animals was performed and eight animals were randomized to nephrectomy, cryotherapy, or a sham procedure on day 11. By this time point tumor-implanted animals would naturally have developed metastases. The median survival of the animals was shown to be 27, 26, and 34.5 days for those treated with sham, nephrectomy, and cryoablation, respectively. This model suggests that cryoablative therapy may provide a survival advantage over nephrectomy in advanced renal cancer. More work needs to be done to elucidate the method of cryotherapy in possibly slowing the fatal progression of metastatic disease.

SELECTION CRITERIA FOR PERCUTANEOUS RENAL CRYOABLATION

Traditionally, nephron-sparing surgery (NSS) has been advocated for tumors less than 4 cm in situations where there is a solitary kidney, renal insufficiency, or a hereditary kidney cancer syndrome, such as VHL, in order to preserve renal function without compromising cancer cure. Recently, these criteria have been expanded to include patients with a normal contralateral kidney. In a retrospective study, Zincke and colleagues[18] showed that individuals undergoing nephrectomy for renal cancer had a 22% chance of developing renal insufficiency (i.e. creatinine >2.0 mg/dl) versus a 12% rate among patients who had only a nephron-sparing approach; patients were followed for >10 years. However, despite this higher level of renal insufficiency, in another study the incidence of renal dialysis was similar between patients with a partial or total nephrectomy. Of note, at 10 years the chance of a local recurrence was 1% in the nephrectomy group and 5% in the partial nephrectomy cohort.[19]

Accordingly, in keeping with the open NSS indications, in the series on percutaneous cryoablation the size criterion has generally been tumors less than 4 cm and usually less than 3 cm so that only one or at most two cryoprobes would be needed. The range of a 5-mm cryoprobe is 2.2×4.4 cm to obtain a temperature of $-40°C$ or 2.9×5.1 cm to obtain a temperature of $-20°C$ (e.g. Endocare Inc., Irvine, CA) and a 17-gauge (1.47-mm) probe has a $-20°C$ range of 2.45×3.6 cm and $-40°C$ of 1.45×3.4 cm (Ice Rod, Oncura, Plymouth Meeting, PA).

PERCUTANEOUS RENAL CRYOABLATION: CLINICAL EXPERIENCE

Percutaneous renal cryoablation was first reported by Uchida et al[20] using ultrasound guidance and a liquid nitrogen system. A 6.8-mm probe was used to obtain a $-20°C$ temperature for 5 minutes. This was following pre-procedure renal artery embolization. The two patients treated already had metastatic disease; they succumbed 5 and 10 months after treatment, though improved Karnofsky status, tumor necrosis, and tumor shrinkage were observed.

Since then, Shingleton[21] has employed magnetic resonance image guidance to perform percutaneous renal cryoablation. This author's experience was published in 2001[21] and included 20 patients with 22 lesions ranging from 1.8 to 7 cm. Typically, two to four 17-gauge cryoprobes (Oncura, Plymouth Meeting, PA) were used with three freeze–thaw cycles achieving a minimum tissue temperature of $-40°C$. Only one patient in this series had persistent tumor requiring retreatment. This series now includes 90 patients and 111 lesions treated over a 4-year period; this includes treatment of 21 patients with a solitary kidney. A 92% overall success rate at median follow-up of 30 months has been reported.[22] Shingleton has also reported this technique in patients with Von Hippel–Lindau disease and for treating tumors in a transplanted kidney.[23,24] In this author's overall experience there were nine complications of which one was a major perinephric hemorrhage requiring transfusion. With an average follow-up of 2.5 years (1–4 years), no patient has developed metastatic disease and the cancer-specific survival has been 100%. Of note, 13% of patients required re-treatments; none of these proceeded to partial or radical nephrectomy.

Harada et al[25] have also described their technique of percutaneous renal cryoablation using open coil magnetic resonance image guidance. This group treated four patients with an average lesion size of 2.5 cm and documented resolution of the tumors and the safety of the technique. The argon-based Cryohit system by Oncura was also used in this group with 2- or 3-mm cryoprobes to administer two freeze–thaw cycles.

In 2004 Bassignani et al[26] reported their initial pilot experience with real-time ultrasound-guided percutaneous renal cryoablation using six to eleven, 17-gauge cryoprobes. They treated three patients with four masses in four kidneys. Lesions ranged from 3 to 6.2 cm. Follow-up CT or MRI at 6–7 weeks showed absence of enhancement and a 63% ± 15% shrinkage of the treated lesion without enhancement.

Gupta et al[27] have reported their experience with percutaneous cryoablation under CT fluoroscopic guidance in 20 patients (27 tumors); 11 patients (16 tumors) had a mean follow-up of 8 months. An argon-based system was used to administer two freeze–thaw cycles of 10–12 minutes each via a 2.3-mm cryoprobe. The mean tumor size was 2.5 cm with five of the tumors being central and 11 non-central. Fifteen of the 16 lesions with follow-up showed no enhancement; the one lesion with persistent enhancement was large and centrally located. There was one hemorrhagic complication requiring transfusion in a patient with a large central tumor.

TECHNIQUE OF PERCUTANEOUS RENAL CRYOABLATION USING MAGNETIC RESONANCE IMAGING GUIDANCE

The technique of percutaneous cryoablation using magnetic resonance imaging guidance has been described and demonstrated in video format by Shingleton.[21] Their technique is outlined here and uses the 17-gauge argon-based Cryohit system by Oncura.

Following fulfillment of selection criteria (i.e. no pacemaker or other contraindication to MRI, absence of bleeding diathesis), patients are evaluated by physical examination, chest radiography, electrocardiogram, serum electrolyte panel, complete blood count, and coagulation profile. The procedure is performed after the induction of a general anesthetic. Arterial and central lines were placed for intraoperative monitoring in this series, though with the low rate of perinephric hemorrhage requiring transfusion (one patient of 90 treated), these may not be necessary unless co-morbidities or anesthetic concerns dictate otherwise. A Foley catheter is also inserted. Prone positioning is optimal and this is achieved on an open interventional MRI docking table. The patient is then advanced into the magnetic bore and axial fast-spin echo images are obtained to localize the mass.

Following identification of the ideal probe entry site, the skin is prepared and draped in the usual sterile fashion. The skin can then be anesthetized with 1% Xylocaine and epinephrine and a 17-gauge probe, 15 cm in length, of MRI-compatible construct (titanium) within its sheath is inserted. Axial fast-spin echo images at two images per second are used to monitor the probe as it advances to the lesion. A breath-hold technique can also be used to acquire images in the axial, coronal, and sagittal planes to obtain a better spatial definition and minimize probe artifact.

The probe is then advanced through the center of the mass until the tip lies at the distal inner border. If the tumor is anterior, the probe is directed through the parenchyma and away from the collecting system. The probe should not traverse the collecting system. Anterior lesions must not be abutting the duodenum or large bowel. The cryosystem is then activated to −190°C for a 10-minute freeze and the growing iceball is monitored frequently to avoid injury to the collecting system and surrounding structures. The iceball, represented on T-1 imaging by a signal void, is allowed to advance until the entire lesion is enveloped and a 5-mm margin is noted surrounding the tumor. If the size or configuration of the mass is such that the targeted volume cannot be covered, thawing and repositioning with an overlapping technique is used to try to achieve complete tumor ablation. In this regard, two to four probes are typically used to treat the desired volume. Three freeze–thaw cycles are performed.

After the third cycle the probe is removed and the sheath packed with absorbable hemostatic material such as gelatin pledgets or oxidized regenerated cellulose. The patient is then extubated and an overnight stay in hospital with the Foley catheter *in situ* is recommended. The average treatment time is 79 minutes. Complete blood count and electrolytes are checked on the following day. Follow-up of the cryolesion with MRI or CT scan at 1 week and 1, 3, 6, 12, 18, and 24 months and then annually is recommended. However, at this time, most clinicians are skipping the 1-week and 1-month study as this can be unreliable and instead are waiting to initiate follow-up studies at 3 months after treatment (Table 10.1).

TECHNIQUE OF PERCUTANEOUS RENAL CRYOABLATION USING REAL-TIME ULTRASOUND GUIDANCE

The technique of percutaneous cryoablation using ultrasound guidance has been described by Bassignani and Theodorescu and associates at the University of Virginia Health Sciences Center. This pilot study of three patients with four lesions employed a Philips ATL HDI 5000 ultrasound unit and a 3-MHz transducer with an attached needle guide (Philips ATL Ultrasound, Bothell, Washington). One patient had biopsy-proven renal cell carcinoma and the second patient had a known contralateral renal cell carcinoma, which had been resected 18 months prior. The third patient did not have histological confirmation of malignancy. The cryosurgical unit employed was the Cryohit system by Oncura. Prior to the procedure, each lesion had to be visible in its entirety with ultrasound via the flank or back and this determined optimum positioning as well as candidacy for the treatment.

All patients received a general anesthetic and were positioned prone with either a pillow under the abdomen or the table flexed. A 17-gauge temperature-monitoring needle was placed with the tip advanced 1–2 mm beyond the border of the mass. A specifically designed template containing two concentric rings with guide holes

Table 10.1   Expected lesion shrinkage post percutaneous cryotherapy

Time post percutaneous cryoablation (months)	Percentage decrease in size
3	22
6	28
12	50
18	70
24	70
36	67

WB Shingleton et al. 2004 (personal communication).

spaced exactly 1 cm apart was used to place six to 11 needles equidistant from each other into the lesion.

Two freeze cycles were then applied for an average of 10 minutes each followed by 10 minutes of active thawing. The leading edge of the iceball is carefully monitored and a leading margin of the iceball 1 cm beyond the mass is the goal. The average operating room time was 2 hours and 17 minutes.

Patients were hospitalized overnight. No significant changes in renal function, as measured by serum creatinine, were recorded even though one patient had a solitary kidney and chronic renal insufficiency at baseline. CT or MRI was performed at follow-up after 6–7 weeks.

TECHNIQUE OF PERCUTANEOUS RENAL CRYOABLATION USING REAL-TIME CT FLUOROSCOPIC GUIDANCE

CT fluoroscopy is a technique initially described in 1994 by Katada et al[28-30] which uses low-milliampere second and partial reconstruction algorithms to enable the acquisition of lower-resolution images by using either intermittent or continuous fluoroscopy. This permits accurate guidance of the needle with the elegance of real-time ultrasound or X-ray fluoroscopy.

At the University of California, Irvine, percutaneous cryoablation using CT fluoroscopy has been used to treat three patients with renal lesions. The cryosurgical unit employed probes of 2-mm diameter (Endocare, Irvine, CA). The patients received a general anesthetic and were positioned prone. In two patients, two probes were placed and in the third, a single probe was used. After imaging the lesion, an 18-gauge Temno coaxial biopsy system (Cardinal Health, Dublin, Ohio) was passed into the targeted lesion; two biopsies were taken for cytology and histopathological analysis. Next, the cryoprobe was positioned in the lesions such that its tip was at the distal-most border of the lesion. Two freeze cycles were then applied for an average of 10 minutes each followed by 10 minutes of active thawing. The leading edge of the iceball is carefully monitored; this edge should extend 5 mm beyond the border of the mass. The average time in the interventional radiology suite was 3 hours. All three lesions were less than 3 cm and pre-procedure biopsies were inconclusive in two and showed an angiomyolipoma in the third patient. At present, all biopsies result in an immediate frozen section reading to provide a proper tissue diagnosis. On follow-up imaging, ranging from 6 to 9 months, all lesions had decreased in size and were without enhancement.

Patients were hospitalized overnight. No significant changes in renal function, as measured by serum creatinine, were recorded. CT was performed at follow-up intervals of 3 months. At 1 year, no retreatment has been necessary.

POST-TREATMENT FOLLOW-UP: IMAGING CHARACTERISTICS

Follow-up with MRI or CT scan in the Shingleton series has typically demonstrated a small rim of peripheral enhancement with absence of central enhancement on imaging performed at 1 week and 1 month. Occasionally, perinephric hemorrhage may preclude optimal visualization of the treated lesion on the early follow-up scans. On imaging at 12 months post-treatment, 13 of 22 masses had decreased in size whereas six masses had disappeared; all masses were non-enhancing. Imaging with CT or MRI was originally recommended at 1 week and 1, 3, 6, and 12 months.[21]

However, because of potential confusion on the early scans due to rim enhancement, hematoma, or lesion swelling, many investigators now recommend delaying initial scans until 3 months in the otherwise asymptomatic patient.

COMPLICATIONS OF PERCUTANEOUS RENAL CRYOTHERAPY

In the 90-patient series of Shingleton,[22] complications were mostly minor: one urinary tract infection, one wound infection, five flank paresthesias, and one patient with respiratory difficulty. There was one major complication, a perinephric hemorrhage requiring transfusion.

If the iceball is not accurately monitored, the potential for engulfing the ureter resulting in ureteropelvic junction stricture and hydronephrosis or injury to the colon and other nearby structures exists and has been described in laboratory models.[31] However, to date, this has not been reported in clinical series. Nonetheless, to decrease the chances of this occurring when treating an anterior or medial lesion, Milner et al[32] described their innovative technique of CT-guided saline mobilization of the colon to facilitate renal cryoablation. In one patient, they essentially created a "salinoma" by using a 22-gauge needle to inject 500 cc of saline between the colon and the tumor prior to the cryoablation. More saline was injected as necessary (determined by intermittent CT) and this provided an effective method of colon mobilization for the procedure. This patient is lesion free on follow-up CT.

It is imperative that the iceball be monitored very closely during its formation, preferably at least every 1 minute during freezing, especially when anteriorly located tumors are being treated. As mentioned in an earlier section, Sung et al[9] Raj et al[11] and Janzen et al[12] have demonstrated the relative resistance of the collecting system to cryosurgical injury and indeed there have been no clinical reports of urine leak, urinoma, or urinary fistula following renal cryoablation. However, one should be cognizant when placing the cryoprobe to avoid direct puncture of the collecting system as this may theoretically increase the risk for the aforementioned complications.

Table 10.2   Probe sizes and −20 and −40°C area of Endocare cryoprobes (Endocare Inc., Irvine, CA)

Probe size (mm)	Area of −20°C (cm)(W × L)	Area of −40°C (cm)(W × L)
1.7	2.1 × 4.2	1.4 × 3.5
2.4	2.8 × 4.8	1.9 × 3.7
3.0	2.4 × 4.5	1.8 × 3.6
5.0	2.9 × 5.1	2.2 × 4.4
8.0	4.2 × 5.7	3.6 × 5.1

Table 10.3   Probe sizes and −20 and −40°C area of Oncura cryoprobes (Oncura, Plymouth Meeting, PA)

Probe type	Probe size (gauge/mm)	Area of −20°C (cm)(W × L)	Area of −40°C (cm)(W × L)	Iceball size (cm)(W × L)
CryoNeedle	17/1.47	1.38 × 1.74	0.82 × 1.64	1.8 × 2.7
IceRod	17/1.47	2.45 × 3.6	1.45 × 3.4	3.2 × 5.6

Table 10.4 Summary of clinical series of open, laparoscopic, and percutaneous renal

Mode	Authors	Number of patients	Length of follow-up	Number of recurrences	Number of retreatments	Secondary procedures	Cancer-specific survival
Open	Delworth et al 1996[36]	2 (2 RCC; 1 AML)	1–3 months	0	0	0	100
	Rodriguez et al 2000[37]	4 open 3 lap.	Mean 14.2 months (0.1–28.5)	0	0	0	100
	Khorsandi et al 2002[38]	17	Median 30 months (10–60)	0	0	0	100
	Rukstalis et al 2001[39]	29	Median 16 months (1–43)	1	1	0	100
Laparoscopic	Harmon et al 2004[40]	120	1996–2003	6	1	2 lap radical nephrectomies; 1 HAL partial; 1 observation	100
	Hasan et al 2004[41]	40	48 months	2	0	2 (radical nephrectomy)	100
	Lee et al 2003[42]	20	Mean 14.2 months (1–40)	0	0	0	100
	Nadler et al 2003[43]	15	147–716 days	1	0	1 (radical nephrectomy for multifocal disease)	100
	Colon et al 2003[44]	8	Mean 11.8 months (5–16)	0	0	0	100
Percutaneous	Gupta et al 2005[27]	20	Mean 8 months				
	Shingleton et al 2004[22]	90	Median 30 months (range 12–48)		13%	0	100
	Bassignani et al 2004[26]	3 (4 masses)	Range 3–13 months	0	0	0	100
	Harada et al 2001[25]	4	Not stated	1	1	0	100
	Uchida et al 1995[20]	2 with metastatic RCC	5 and 10 months	0	0	0	0

cryoablation								
Tumor size (cm)	Number of freezes	Number of probes	Size of probe	Cryogen employed	OR time	Hospital stay	Imaging technique	Development of metastases
2–3 cm; 7 × 10 cm	Double	3	3 mm	Liquid nitrogen	210–270 minutes	2–5 days	US	0
Mean 2.2 cm (1.8–3.0)	Double (5); single (2)	1	3 mm		Mean 234 minutes (range 205–266)	Mean 4.4 days (range 3–8)	US	0
2.0 cm (1.1–4.2)	Double	1–4	3 mm/ 8 mm		180 minutes (range 135–255)	Median 2 days (range 2–8)	US	0
2.2 cm (1.0–4.7)	Double	1–3	3 mm/ 8 mm	Liquid nitrogen (27); argon (2)		3 days (2–11); 4 days (2–8)*	US	0
–	–	–	–	–	–	–	–	0
Mean 2.4 cm	Double	1	4.8 mm	Argon	174 minutes (range 60–270)	Mean 1.8 days (range 1–5)	US	0
Range 1.4–4.5 cm	Double	1	4.8 mm		305 minutes (range 155–715)	2.6 days (range 1–9)	US	0
Mean 2.15 cm (range 1.2–3.2)	Double	1	4.8 mm	Liquid nitrogen	Mean 260 minutes	Mean 3.5 days (range 1–11)	US	0
Mean 2.6 cm (range 1.4–3.8)	Double	1	3 mm	Argon	Mean 120 ± 27.8 minutes	Mean 2.9 ± 1.6 days	US	0
Mean 2.5 cm	Double		2.3 mm	Argon			CT	
<5 cm	Triple	2–4	17-gauge	Argon	78 minutes	Overnight	MRI	0
Mean 2.5 ± 1.2 cm	Double	6–11	17-gauge	Argon	Mean 137 ± 20 minutes	Overnight	US	0
Mean 2.5 cm (range 2–3)	Double	2–4	2 or 3 mm	Argon	Mean 120 minutes (range 90–150)	1 day (3)	MRI	0
			6.8 mm			7 days (1)	US	Both presented with mets

Warlick et al[33] presented data on known radiographic iceball extension into the collecting system during percutaneous CT-guided cryoablation in eight patients treated at Johns Hopkins. All tumors extended to within 9 mm of the collecting system and one to five cryoprobes were employed. In six patients the iceball extended into the collecting system and in the other two patients, to within 3 mm and 5 mm. No patients developed evidence of a leak or fistula, once again confirming the safety of cryoablation in close proximity to the collecting system.

DEVICES AND PROBES CURRENTLY IN CLINICAL USE

There are currently two cryotherapy companies supplying probes for renal lesions: Endocare and Oncura.

The Cryocare CS system by Endocare has been marketed for the treatment of prostate cancer and these same probes are also being used for renal cryotherapy. Argon gas is again employed as the cryogen. Available probe sizes and the area of the $-20°C$ isotherm are shown in Table 10.2. Rewcastle et al[34] evaluated the 3.4-mm CRYOprobe by Endocare and were able to devise a simulated time-dependent model for predicting the volume encompassed by critical isotherms and cited that this model should be used to ensure that the anticipated volume had indeed been treated (Table 10.2).

The Cryohit system (Table 10.3), by Oncura, is the system employed by Shingleton and associates in their series. The system utilizes 17-gauge (1.47-mm) probes to deliver argon gas to the probe tip through an inner lumen and then this is depressurized via a ball valve mechanism to the outer lumen where the gas is carried up the probe and away from the treated area. Freezing temperatures of -175 to $-190°C$ at the probe tip are reached by depressurizing the argon gas (Joule-Thompson effect). Pressurized helium gas is used to effect thawing and temperatures up to 70°C. In this system, all probes are single-use and MRI-compatible (titanium construction).

The Seed Net system (Table 10.3), also by Oncura, and employed for prostate cryosurgery is also being marketed for renal cryoablation. This system uses 17-gauge titanium IceRod probes which are closed-tip, thin-walled needles containing a 0.4-mm heat exchanger and a copper/nickel cryogenic Joule-Thompson assembly. These probes have a tear-drop or elliptical tip configuration. Ames et al[35] recently evaluated these novel cryoprobes in a pig model, and found that the -20 and $-40°C$ isotherms were comparable to the larger standard probes and also to three standard CryoNeedle 17-gauge probes inserted by template. These novel probes will likely further facilitate percutaneous renal cryoablation by minimizing the number of needles required and reducing the potential for hemorrhage due to multiple punctures.

FUTURE DIRECTIONS

The use of MRI guidance for percutaneous procedures requires collaboration between urologists and interventional radiologists. Total procedure costs are high due to the imaging modality. Many urologists, however, are adept with the use of ultrasound, specifically for prostate biopsy and prostate cryotherapy. The application of these sonographic skills to renal imaging and procedures is truly within the realm of urology. After perfection of the technique, such procedures as renal cryoablation could be performed as outpatient or office procedures under intravenous sedation, permitting early discharge after a brief period of observation, without compromising safety. Much work remains to be done in this area, but the fact that to date no reported patient has developed either metastatic disease or succumbed to renal cancer following cryotherapy is encouraging. The immunologic impact of this therapy also needs to be further elucidated. However, in the final analysis, the proof of efficacy will be in the follow-up and final judgment awaits 5-year data (Table 10.4).

REFERENCES

1. Arnott J. On the Treatment of Cancer by the Regulated Application of an Anesthetic Temperature. London: J Churchill, 1851.
2. Soanes WA, Gonder MJ, Shulman S. Apparatus and technique for cryosurgery of the prostate. J Urol 1966; 96: 508–11.
3. Flocks RH, Nelson CM, Boatman DL. Perineal cryosurgery for prostatic carcinoma. J Urol 1972; 108: 933–5.
4. Long JP, Faller GT. Percutaneous cryoablation of the kidney in a porcine model. Cryobiology 1999; 38: 89–93.
5. Onik GM, Reyes G, Cohen JK, Porterfield B. Ultrasound characteristics of renal cryosurgery. Urology 1993; 42: 212–15.
6. Nakada SY, Jerde TJ, Lee FT, Warner T. Efficacy of cryoblation and nephrectomy in treating implanted VX-2 carcinoma in rabbit kidneys. J Urol 2000; 163: 10. Abstract.
7. Shingleton WB, Farabaugh P, Hughson M, Sewell PK. Percutaneous cryoablation of porcine kidneys with magnetic resonance imaging monitoring. J Urol 2001; 166: 289–91.
8. Wooley ML, Schulsinger DA, Durand DB et al. Effect of freezing parameters (freeze cycle and thaw process) on tissue destruction following renal cryoablation. J Endourol 2002; 16: 519–22.
9. Sung GT, Gill IS, Hsu TH et al. Effect of intentional cryo-injury to the renal collecting system. J Urol 2003; 170: 619–22.
10. Rehman J, Landman J, Lee D et al. Needle based ablation of renal parenchyma using microwave, cryoablation, impedance- and temperature-based monopolar and bipolar radiofrequency, and liquid and gel chemoablation: Laboratory studies and review of the literature. J Endourol 2004; 18: 83–104.
11. Brashears JH 3rd, Raj GV, Crisci A et al. Renal cryoablation and radio frequency ablation: an evaluation of worst case scenarios in a porcine model. J Urol 2005; 173: 2160–5.
12. Janzen NK, Perry KT, Han K-R et al. The effects of intentional cryoablation and radiofrequency ablation of renal tissue involving the collecting system in a porcine model. J Urol 2005; 173: 1368–74.
13. Gage AA, Baust J. Mechanisms of tissue injury in cryosurgery. Cryobiology 1998; 37: 171–86.
14. Hoffman NE, Bischof JC. The cryobiology of cryosurgical injury. Urology 2002; 60 (Suppl 1): 40–9.
15. Baust J, Gage AA, Ma H, Zhang CM. Minimally invasive cryosurgery – technological advances. Cryobiology 1997; 34(4): 373–84.
16. Chosy SG, Nakada SY, Lee FT, Warner TF. Monitoring renal cryosurgery: predictors of tissue necrosis in swine. J Urol 1998; 159: 1370–4.
17. Hedican SP, Wilkinson ER, Lee FT, Warner TF et al. Cryoablation of advanced renal cancer has survival advantages in a murine model compared to nephrectomy. J Urol 2004; 171: 206. Abstract.
18. Lau WKO, Blute ML, Weaver AL et al. Matched comparison of radical nephrectomy vs nephron sparing surgery in patients with unilateral renal cell carcinoma and a normal contralateral kidney. Mayo Clin Proc 2000; 75: 1236–42.
19. Corman JM, Penson DF, Hur K et al. Comparison of complications after radical and partial nephrectomy: results from the National Veterans Administration Surgical Quality Improvement Program. BJU Int 2000; 86(7): 782–9.

20. Uchida M, Imaide Y, Sugimoto K et al. Percutaneous cryosurgery for renal tumours. BJU 1995; 75: 132–7.
21. Shingleton WB, Sewell PE. Percutaneous renal tumor cryoablation with magnetic resonance imaging guidance. J Urol 2001; 165: 773–6.
22. Shingleton WB, Sewell PE. Percutaneous renal cryoablation: results in the first 90 patients. J Urol 2004; 171: 463. Abstract.
23. Shingleton WB, Sewell PE. Percutaneous renal cryoablation of renal tumors in patients with Von-Hippel–Lindau disease. J Urol 2002; 167: 1268–70.
24. Shingleton WB, Sewell PE. Percutaneous cryoablation of renal cell carcinoma in a transplanted kidney. BJU Int 2002; 90: 137–8.
25. Harada J, Dohi M, Mogami T et al. Initial experience of percutaneous renal cryosurgery under the guidance of a horizontal open MRI system. Radiat Med 2001; 19: 291–6.
26. Bassignani MJ, Moore Y, Watson L, Theodorescu D. Pilot experience with real-time ultrasound guided percutaneous renal mass cryoablation. J Urol 2004; 171: 1620–23.
27. Gupta A, Allaf ME, Warlick CA et al. Percutaneous renal tumor cryoablation under CT guidance: initial clinical experience. J Urol 2005; 173: 413. Abstract.
28. Katada K, Anno H, Ogura Y et al. Early clinical experience with real-time CT fluoroscopy. Nippon Acta Radiol 1994; 54: 1172–4.
29. Paulson EK, Sheafor DH, Enterline DS et al. CT fluoroscopy-guided interventional procedures: techniques and radiation dose to radiologists. Radiology 2001; 220: 161–7.
30. Wagner AL. CT-fluoroscopic guided cervical nerve root blocks. Am J Neuroradiol 2005; 26: 43–4.
31. Campbell SC, Krishnamurthi V, Chow G et al. Renal cryosurgery: experimental evaluation of treatment parameters. Urology 1998; 52: 29–34.
32. Milner J, Borge M, Sharma S et al. Percutaneous CT guided saline mobilization of the colon to facilitate renal cryoablation. J Urol 2005; 173: 320. Abstract.
33. Warlick CA, Lima GC, Allaf ME et al. Collecting system involvement during renal tumor cryoablation. J Urol 2005; 173: 263. Abstract.
34. Rewcastle JC, Sandison GA, Hahn LJ et al. A model for the time-dependent thermal distribution within an iceball surrounding a cryoprobe. Phys Med Biol 1998; 43: 3519–34.
35. Ames CD, Vanlangendonk R, Venkatesh R et al. Enhanced renal parenchymal cryoablation with novel 17-gauge cryoprobes. Urology 2004; 64: 173–5.
36. Delworth DG, Pisters LL, Fornage BD, von Eschenbach AC. Cryotherapy for renal cell carcinoma and angiomyolipoma. J Urol 1996; 155: 252–5.
37. Rodriguez R, Chan DY, Bishoff JT et al. Renal ablative cryosurgery in selected patients with peripheral renal masses. Urology 2000; 55: 25–30.
38. Khorsandi M, Foy RC, Chong W et al. Preliminary experience with cryoablation of renal lesions smaller than 4 cm. J Am Osteopath Assoc 2002; 102: 277–81.
39. Rukstalis DB, Khorsandi M, Garcia FU et al. Clinical experience with open renal cryoablation. Urology 2001; 57: 34–9.
40. Harmon JD, Parulkar BG, Doble A, Rukstalis DB. Critical assessment of cancer recurrence following renal cryoablation: a multi-center review. J Urol 2004; 171: 469. Abstract.
41. Hasan W, Gill I, Spaliviero M et al. Renal cryoablation: 4-year follow-up. J Urol 2004; 171: 438. Abstract.
42. Lee DI, McGinnis DE, Feld R, Strup SE. Retroperitoneal laparoscopic cryoablation of small renal tumors: intermediate results. Urology 2003; 61: 83–8.
43. Nadler RB, Kim SC, Rubenstein JN et al. Laparoscopic renal cryosurgery: the Northwestern experience. J Urol 2003; 170: 1121–5.
44. Colon I, Fuchs GJ. Early experience with laparoscopic cryoablation in patients with small renal tumors and severe comorbidities. J Endourol 2003; 17: 415–23.

11

Renal ablation: comparison of cryoablation and radiofrequency

C. Charles Wen, Stephen Y. Nakada

Background and introduction • Background and technique: cryoablation • Background and technique: RFA • Access • Outcomes • Complications • Comment

BACKGROUND AND INTRODUCTION

The use of nephron-sparing surgery for renal cancer dates back to 1887 when Czerny performed the first partial nephrectomy. In 1969 Robson challenged the role of partial nephrectomies, making radical nephrectomy the gold standard.[1] It was not until the early 1980s when the increased detection of incidental low-stage tumors through the widespread use of renal imaging led to the re-popularization of nephron-sparing surgery.[2,3] As the long-term outcomes from partial nephrectomy confirmed the efficacy of nephron-sparing surgery, less-invasive ablative techniques were developed in efforts to achieve the benefits of minimally invasive procedures. Currently, the two most published ablation techniques are cryoablation and radio-frequency ablation (RFA).[4]

Present-day indications for renal tumor ablation mirror those for partial nephrec-tomy. Selection criteria include tumors less than 4 cm, tumors in functionally solitary kidneys and bilateral synchronous tumor syndromes, and patients with multiple asynchronous tumors.[1,5,6] Primarily we treat enhancing solid tumors, with a minimum enhancement of 15–20 Hounsfield units (HU) on CT, or enhancement with gadolin-ium MRI.[7] Although the gap between the indications for ablative procedures and partial nephrectomies is narrowing, the low morbidity and quicker recovery time of ablative therapies make them appealing compared to partial nephrectomy, particu-larly in patients with significant comorbidities and shorter life expectancy.[8,9]

Relative contraindications to ablation include renal tumors that are contiguous with bowel, ureter, or large vessels, and tumors abutting the collecting system.[7,10] Relative contraindications to performing laparoscopic access for ablation include prior abdominal or renal surgery and history of renal inflammation.[8] Most authors believe that tumors on the anterior or medial aspect of the kidney should be consid-ered contraindications to percutaneous ablation, and favor approaching these tumors laparoscopically.[11] However, in Shingleton et al's series, 20% of the tumors ablated percutaneously were anterior.[12] None of the tumors were adjacent to bowel or col-lecting system and a slow freeze technique with 1 minute of freezing followed by imaging to assess iceball to bowel distance was used. In addition, MRI was the primary imaging modality, making it possible to image beyond the iceball, where if ultrasound was used, shadowing would prevent accurate determination of iceball

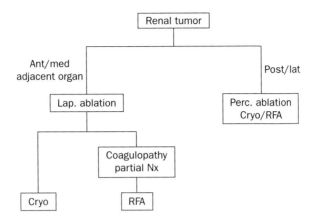

Figure 11.1   Renal tumor ablation algorithm.

progression on the distal edge. Under these circumstances a percutaneous technique may be considered for anterior tumors.

Currently, there are no standard guidelines for choosing between cryoablation and radiofrequency ablation; however, it has been shown in animal models that cryoablation has a decreased risk for collecting system injury, whereas RFA appears to have a lower rate of significant hemorrhage.[13–15] In addition, RFA is better suited for exophytic tumors likely due to the insulating effect of the fat surrounding the lesion, while endophytic tumors treated with RFA may have a higher incidence of collecting-system injuries and inferior outcomes.[7] These differences are not as evident with cryoablation.

There are also no guidelines for choosing a laparoscopic versus percutaneous approaches; however, it is generally accepted that medial and anterior lesions are best served by laparoscopic access to the tumor.[15] A treatment algorithm for ablation therapy can be seen in Figure 11.1. Another indication for choosing a laparoscopic approach is when an ablative procedure is combined with excision of a lesion, as reported by Cadeddu and co-workers performing RF-assisted laparoscopic partial nephrectomy.[15]

BACKGROUND AND TECHNIQUE: CRYOABLATION

Percutaneous renal cryosurgery was first reported by Uchida et al in 1995 for two patients with high-stage renal cancers.[16] Since then, cryoablation has been performed with open access and laparoscopic access.[17,18] Cryoablation relies on the principle that temperatures below −20–40°C are needed to induce cell death. The mechanism of this cell death is twofold. First, there is direct mechanical cellular injury from ice crystal formation within and around the cells. Secondly, vascular injury after thawing results in microcirculatory failure, depriving the surrounding tissue of blood. This results in a necrotic zone, which becomes evident approximately 2 days after therapy.[19] Recent work has revealed a possible third mechanism of cell death based on increased rates of apoptosis in the peripheral zone of the necrotic lesion.[20]

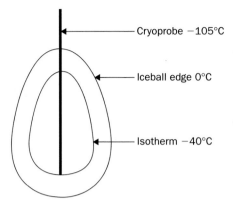

Cryoprobe −105°C

Iceball edge 0°C

Isotherm −40°C

Figure 11.2 Cryoprobe isotherm. From the cryoprobe to the iceball edge, temperature contin-ues to rise in a predictable pattern. The −40°C isotherm should completely cover the tumor in order to ensure proper ablation.

Renal cryoablation was initially performed with liquid nitrogen (−195.8°C). However, continued iceball progression after halting the liquid nitrogen perfusion made controlling the iceball size difficult. Pressurized argon gas (−185.7°C) elimi-nated this delay between the end of infusion and iceball progression. Other advances in cryoablation include smaller probe sizes, larger iceball to probe size ratios, allow-ing for smaller probes to be used, and insulated probe shafts, which limit the amount of cooling proximal to the tip.

Cryoprobes currently range in size from 1.7 mm to 8 mm. Percutaneous cryo-probes range from 1.7 to 2.4 mm whereas laparoscopic probes range from 3 to 8 mm. Probe tips are beveled for percutaneous use or blunt for laparoscopic treatments. Probes can create iceball shapes that are oblong or round, and iceball size increases with probe diameter. In order to achieve renal cell death, temperatures must be below −19.4°C. For necrosis of virtually all human tissues −40°C is required.[21,22]

From the edge of the iceball (0°C) to the probe (−185.7°C) the temperatures become progressively lower, making the kill zone smaller than the iceball (Figure 11.2). Therefore, iceball size must exceed that of the tumor in order to ensure that the −19.4°C to −40°C isotherm covers the entire lesion.[22] The distance that the iceball has to extend beyond the tumor margin varies with probe selection and ranges from 3.5 to 6.0 mm for percutaneous probes.

Freezing of a lesion should be done as quickly as possible, and the freeze cycle should be 10 minutes (Figure 11.3). The lesion is then thawed either passively or actively with helium gas. Animal studies have shown that the type of thaw process did not affect tissue damage.[23] This freeze–thaw cycle is then repeated, as the second cycle increases the percent cell death within the original iceball without extending the frozen margin and risking unnecessary injury to adjacent structures. After a passive or active (He) second thaw the cryoprobe can be removed, and if large-diameter (≤5 mm) probes are used during a laparoscopic approach, hemostatic agents such as fibrin glue, Surgicel, or Floseal can be used in the cryoprobe track. When using Floseal, it is valuable to wait until the tract thaws enough so that there is some bleeding, as Floseal is more active in this circumstance.

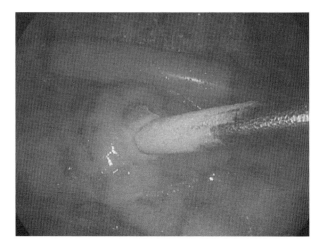

Figure 11.3   Laparoscopic-assisted cryoablation of an exophytic renal lesion. Laparoscopic ultrasound probe behind the lesion monitors the iceball growth. (See also color plate.)

BACKGROUND AND TECHNIQUE: RFA

Radiofrequency ablation for renal tumors was first reported by Zlotta in 1997.[24] Radiofrequency energy is delivered to tissues using specially designed needles that selectively heat only around the needle tip. The tissues are heated to 105°C. At this temperature cell death and coagulation necrosis is expected.[7] After 24–48 hours a necrotic lesion begins to form and at around 7 days it reaches maximum size.[25] The ablated tissue is eventually replaced by fibrosis or is re-absorbed.

Today, there are a multitude of RFA probes available to the practicing urologist (Table 11.1). RFA probes can be monopolar, with energy traveling from the probe tip to a grounding pad, or bipolar with energy traveling from one probe tip to another. RFA can also be performed in a wet environment (virtual electrode) by infusing highly conductive electrolyte solutions to increase the size and speed of ablation without tissue desiccation. RFA probes can be a single electrode that controls tissue coagulation based on time and impedance feedback. Probes may also have an electrode with multiple thermosensing tines that determine the coagulation end points. Some probes are internally cooled by circulating ice-cold saline around the electrode to draw away unwanted heat that is radiated back along the probe. Cooling also limits the charring around the electrode tip, which can cause increased tissue impedance and decreased energy transfer to the edge of the heat ball.[26]

Because real-time ultrasound monitoring is not feasible with RFA, the kill zone estimation is based on minimum activated time and the deployed diameter if using thermosensing tines. The maximum lesion size is not changed by activating the probe for longer periods of time; therefore, it is imperative that the probe be accurately placed into the center of the lesion.[15]

Once the probe is in place and the target temperature is achieved the tissue is heated for 3–8 minutes depending on lesion size. At 50°C, proteins begin to denature, lipids melt, and irreversible tissue destruction tends to occur. At 100°C tissue coagulation, desiccation, and charring takes place.[26] Probe temperatures approach

	Probe type	Probe size	Sensor	Wet/dry	Generator
RITA	Coaxial Christmas tree tines	14–15G	Thermocoupled tines	Dry RFA or hypertonic saline-infused	200 W, 150 W
Radiotherapeutics	Equidistant umbrella tines	14–15G	Impedence	Dry RFA	200 W, 90 W
Radionics	Singe probe	17.5G	Impedence	Dry RFA, internal saline cooling	200 W
Berchtold	Singe probe	14–16G	Impedence	Normal saline-infused	50 W

Table 11.1 Radiofrequency ablation systems

105°C in the center and diminish toward the edge as impedance increases. Heating time algorithms are dependent upon the particular electrode used as well as the electrosurgical generator which can range from 50 to 200 W. For larger lesions a combination of longer heating times and multiple electrodes can be used to ensure adequate kill zone coverage of the tumor.

ACCESS

Both cryoablation and radiofrequency ablation can be done either percutaneously or via laparoscopic access to the tumor. The percutaneous approach can be done with local anesthesia and conscious sedation whereas general anesthesia is required for laparoscopy.

For percutaneous access the patient is placed in prone position with a Foley catheter. Renal biopsy can be performed prior to starting the ablation. Sterile water can be injected into the paranephric space prior to RFA, to prevent injury to adjacent organs.[27] An ultrasonic probe with a renal biopsy guide can be used to direct the cryoprobe or the RFA electrode into the center of the renal lesion. MRI or CT fluoroscopy can be used intermittently to assess RFA lesion progress whereas cryolesions can be monitored real time with ultrasound.[10,28]

With cryoablation, multiple cryoprobes can be placed into the same lesion to increase iceball diameter. For RFA there are currently no commercially available devices to allow for multiple probe placement. When the ablation is completed, probes are removed and patients should be observed for hemostasis and pain. Postoperative hematocrit is recommended.

The laparoscopic access to renal tumors for ablative procedures is similar to that of laparoscopic partial nephrectomy. A transperitoneal approach can be used for all tumors whereas a retroperitoneal approach should be reserved for posterior/posterolateral tumors. When using the transperitoneal approach the patient is placed in a lateral decubitus position with a Foley catheter. At our institution a Veress needle is placed midway between the umbilicus and the superior iliac crest, lateral to the rectus muscle. This is also the site for the first trocar. A second port is placed at the lateral margin of the umbilicus and the third port is placed in a subcostal position, just lateral to midline, half way between the xiphoid and the umbilicus. The colon is reflected medially, and Gerota's fascia is dissected off the kidney around the tumor. A renal biopsy is obtained at this time. Intraoperative laparoscopic ultrasound can be used to identify the lesion and determine accurate lesion depths. When performing cryoablation, the 5-mm blunt-tip cryoprobe can be inserted through one of the trochars and directed into the renal tumor. During ablation, constant monitoring of the cryoprobe and electrode will prevent accidental injury to adjacent structures. Care should also be taken when freezing the tumor to avoid freezing and cracking the trochar. For RFA a percutaneous access may be easier. After the ablation is completed the probe is removed and hemostatic agents can be placed directly into the track. Fascial closures are performed for all 10-mm ports while 5-mm ports only require skin closure. The patient is usually admitted and observed for hemostasis and pain control.

OUTCOMES

Currently there is no standard method for postoperative follow-up after renal tumor ablation. Follow-up schemes designed for partial nephrectomies would not be applicable as most do not recommend follow-up imaging for stage T1 tumors; however, the majority of ablated renal tumors fall into this category. Patients should be evaluated yearly with medical history, physical examination with blood pressure, chest X-ray, serum electrolytes, liver function tests, and renal function tests.[29] The first postoperative imaging should be performed between 3 and 6 months. The ablated lesion should be followed using contrast-enhanced CT or MRI scans. Lack of enhancement on CT or MRI, along with stable or decreased tumor size, is considered a successful ablation. Signs of persistent or recurrent cancer include increased tumor size, lack of tumor shrinkage, nodular or lesion enhancement on MRI, or CT enhancement greater than 10 HU.[7,9,11]

The natural history of post-ablative renal tumors appears to differ between cryoablation and radiofrequency ablation based on postoperative imaging data. Whereas cryoablated lesions tend to shrink over time, lesion treated with radiofrequency ablation vary with some shrinking and others maintaining the original preoperative shape. In addition, cryoablated lesions often exhibit rim enhancement. Bolte et al[30] reported 39% rim enhancement within 3 months with 57% resolution by 14 months.

Longer-term data are becoming available for needle invasive techniques (Tables 11.2 and 11.3). Gill et al[9] reported on 3-year follow-up after cryoablation. They also found rim enhancement after cryoablation was often present up until 3 months after ablation but usually disappeared after that. In their series, 56 patients underwent laparoscopic cryoablation. At 3-year follow-up the average size reduction was 75% and 38% of the cryoablated lesions were undetectable on MRI. Three-year cancer-specific survival rate was 98%. Cestari et al[8] performed laparoscopic cryoablation on 37 patients. At 2-year follow-up 22 of 23 patients had no identifiable lesions on postoperative imaging.

McDougal et al[28] reviewed 4-year follow-up data in 16 patients with renal tumors treated with RFA. They found that several patients had increased tumor size at 3-month follow-up but that successfully treated tumors would subsequently shrink in time. Matsumoto et al[11] studied the evolution of renal tumors after temperature-based

Table 11.2 Cryoablation outcomes

Article	No. of patients	Tumor size ave (cm)	Tumor size range (cm)	Imaging	Approach	Follow-up time	Success rate (%)
Gill[9]	56	2.3	1–5	U/A	Lap	3 years	94
Cestari[8]	37	2.57	1–6	U/S	Lap	20 months ave	95
Nadler[33]	15	2.15	1.2–3.2	U/S	Lap	15 months ave	87
Shingleton[10]	14	3.1	1.8–7.0	MRI	Perc	17 months ave	79

Table 11.3 Radiofrequency ablation outcomes

Article	No. of patients	Tumor size ave (cm)	Tumor size range (cm)	Approach	Follow-up time	Success rate (%)
Hwang[7]	17	N/A	1.2–2.8	Perc and lap	1 year median	96
Matsumoto[11]	60	N/A	4 cm max	Perc, lap, open	13 months median	97
McDougal[28]	16	3.2	1.1–7.1	Perc	4 years	94

RFA with routine postoperative CT scan. In 47 exophytic tumors with a median follow-up time of 13.7 months, they found that the RFA defects had a configuration similar to that of the original tumor with minimal shrinkage. Percutaneous-treated tumors often developed a fibrotic rim of fat. Endophytic tumors often retracted from normal perfused parenchymal tissue with fat infiltration surrounding the ablated defect. Their conclusion was that unlike cryoablated lesions, which appear to undergo lesion shrinkage, lesions after RFA do not appear to reabsorb and stable, non-enhancing lesion indicates treatment success.

Histologic analysis of kill zones after radiofrequency ablation has been performed on radical and partial nephrectomy specimens. Matlaga et al[26] performed RFA on eight patients via an open exposure. Following RFA, partial or radical nephrectomies were performed. Histologic analysis revealed complete destruction of tumor, with no skip areas. A rim of necrosis beyond the tumor margin, ranging from 2 to 13 mm, exhibited loss of normal tubular architecture and NADH stains revealed no evidence of viability. Beyond the treatment margin the renal parenchyma appeared undamaged. Jang et al[31] examined histopathology of three patients with recurrent or persistent cancer after cryoablation. These patients underwent further treatment with nephrectomy and the specimens revealed coagulative necrosis, cholesterol crystal formation, dystrophic calcification, and the absence of viable tumor within the cryoablated lesion.

Both cryo- and radiofrequency ablation appear to have minimal effect on renal function. Gill et al compared average pre-op serum creatinine of 1.2 mg/dl with post-op serum creatinine of 1.4 mg/dl and found no significant difference. This held true for patients with chronic renal insufficiency as well finding pre- and post-op serum creatinines to be similar (3.0 and 2.7 mg/dl, respectively).[9,32] Nadler reports pre- and postoperative creatinine levels after laparoscopic cryoablation of 1.25 and 1.36 mg/dl, respectively.[33] Hwang et al report creatinine clearance pre- and post-RFA to be 115 and 102 mg/dl, respectively.[7] Johnson et al did not find any differences in renal function or blood pressure after treating small renal tumors with RFA; however, they did find acute changes in renal function in two patients, one who underwent multiple simultaneous ablations and one who had ablations with concurrent partial nephrectomy.[34]

Long-term data on the outcomes of ablative therapies have only recently been published. There has been some difficulty in determining how to measure clinical success, in part due to the varied findings on postoperative imaging. The utility of using postoperative biopsy has been suggested but does not appear to be routine or necessary. Reported successful ablations measured by cancer persistence or recurrence after single or multiple treatments ranged from 5.4 to 13.3% for cryoablation.[8,9,10,17,33] Tumor-specific survival at 3 years reported by Gill et al was 98%. For radiofrequency ablation, persistence or recurrence after single or multiple treatments ranged from 4.7% to 17%.[7,11,27,34,35] The difficulty in interpreting these data stems from the considerable variation in patient comorbidities and disease stage from one study to the next. In order to accurately evaluate outcomes from ablative therapies it is necessary to compare data from patients with similar characteristics.

COMPLICATIONS

Complications for CA and RFA can be divided into two categories. The first consists of complications related to the laparoscopic access of renal tumors, which is similar to those of comparable procedures such as laparoscopic partial nephrectomy and laparoscopic cyst decortication.[14] The second category includes complications related to the percutaneous access and ablation processes. The most common complication for both CA and RFA in this category is pain or paresthesia at the probe insertion site after percutaneous ablations. In a multi-institutional review of 271 ablative procedures, pain or paresthesia at the probe site accounted for 64% of the complications in percutaneous ablation procedures. This appears to be more common in patients after CA.[14] An explanation for this finding may be related to the fact that early cryoprobes were non-insulated and the entire cryoprobe was cooled, whereas RFA probes are selectively hot at the tip. Although less, RFA probes were not immune from probe site complications. Reasons for this may include direct heat conduction to the inactive portion of the probe, or injury during removal of the hot probe tip. It is expected that complication rates related to probe site pain and paresthesias will continue to decline largely due to the newer instrumentations including insulated cryoprobes and saline-cooled RFA probes. However, care should be taken to avoid injury to sensory nerves at the body surface.

To date, collecting-system injuries have not been reported with cryoablation. Although histologic data reveal that cryoablation can damage the collecting system, animal studies have shown that RFA is more likely to cause collecting-system injuries.[13] There have been a handful of injuries related to the collecting system; these include urine leak,[14,27] caliceal stricture,[36] ureteral obstruction, and bleeds into the collecting system.[14,27]

Other complications appear to be similar between the CA and RFA groups. These include conversion of a laparoscopic procedure to open due to inability to access the tumor, postoperative ileus, hemorrhage, urinary leaks, and fistulas.[14] Other unique complications include one case report of skin metastases from percutaneous RFA procedure,[36] one case of pancreatic injury after retroperitoneal laparoscopic cryoablation,[37] one case of second-degree burn to grounding site with percutaneous RFA, and three cases of transient lumbar neurapraxia after percutaneous RFA.[27] In our experience, we have seen transient neuralgias following percutaneous cryoablation.

COMMENT

Ablative therapies for renal tumors have found a niche in patients who are older with multiple co-morbidities, and available follow-up data seem promising. Both cryoablation and radiofrequency ablation have proven to be effective means for treating small renal cancers at up to 4 years follow-up. The advantages of the ablative techniques mirror those of partial nephrectomies with maximal preservation of renal function. The advantages of using ablative techniques over open and laparoscopic partial nephrectomies are a faster learning curve, easier control of hemostasis, decreased anesthetic requirements, and quicker times to convalescence. While cryoablation has benefits in ultrasound monitoring and fewer collecting system complications, percutaneous RFA is a compelling treatment option in coagulopathic patients. As the technology and experience with renal tumor ablation continue to grow, the precise role of ablative treatments will become clear.

REFERENCES

1. Uzzo RG, Novick AC. Nephron sparing surgery for renal tumors: indications, techniques and outcomes. J Urol 2001; 166: 6–18.
2. Lau WK, Blute ML, Weaver AL et al. Matched comparison of radical nephrectomy vs nephron-sparing surgery in patients with unilateral renal cell carcinoma and a normal contralateral kidney. Mayo Clin Proc 2000; 75: 1236–42.
3. Fergany AF, Hafez KS, Novick AC. Long-term results of nephron sparing surgery for localized renal cell carcinoma: 10-year followup. J Urol 2000; 163: 442–5.
4. Anderson CJ, Havranek EG. Minimally invasive ablative techniques in renal cancer. Br J Urol 2004; 93: 707–9.
5. Lerner SE, Hawkins CA, Blute ML et al. Disease outcome in patients with low stage renal cell carcinoma treated with nephron sparing or radical surgery. J Urol 1996; 155: 1868.
6. Hafez KS, Fergany AF, Novick AC. Nephron sparing surgery for localized renal cell carcinoma: impact of tumor size on patient survival, tumor recurrence and TNM staging. J Urol 1999; 162: 1930.
7. Hwang JJ, Walther MM, Pautler SE et al. Radio frequency ablation of small renal tumors: intermediate results. J Urol 2004; 171: 1814–18.
8. Cestari A, Guazzoni G, Dell'Acqua V et al. Laparoscopic cryoablation of solid renal masses: intermediate term followup. J Urol 2004; 172: 1267–70.
9. Gill IS, Remer EM, Hasan WA et al. Renal cryoablation: outcome at 3 years. J Urol 2005; 173: 1903–7.
10. Shingleton WB, Sewell PE. Cryoablation of renal tumours in patients with solitary kidneys. Br J Urol 2003; 92: 237–9.
11. Matsumoto ED, Watumull L, Johnson DB et al. The radiographic evolution of radio frequency ablated renal tumors. J Urol 2004; 172: 45–8.

12. Shingleton WB, Sewell PE. Percutaneous renal tumor cryoablation with magnetic resonance imaging guidance. J Urol 2001; 165: 773.

13. Johnson DB, Solomon SB, Su L et al. Defining the complications of cryoablation and radio frequency ablation of small renal tumors: a multi-institutional review. J Urol 2004; 172: 874–7.

14. Brashears JH 3rd, Raj GV, Crisci A et al. Renal cryoablation and radio frequency ablation: an evaluation of worst case scenarios in a porcine model. J Urol 2005; 173: 2160–5.

15. Jacomides L, Ogan K, Watumull L, Cadeddu JA. Laparoscopic application of radio frequency energy enables in situ renal tumor ablation and partial nephrectomy. J Urol 2003; 169: 49–53.

16. Uchida M, Imaide Y, Sugimoto K et al. Percutaneous cryosurgery for renal tumors. Br J Urol 1995; 75: 132.

17. Rukstalis DB, Khorsandi M, Garcia FU et al. Clinical experience with open renal cryoablation. Urology 2001; 57: 34–9.

18. Moon TD, Lee FT, Hedican SP et al. Laparoscopic cryoablation under sonographic guidance for the treatment of small renal tumors. J Endourol 2004; 18: 436–40.

19. Baust JG, Gage AA. The molecular basis of cryosurgery. Br J Urol 2005; 95: 1187–91.

20. Yang WI, Addona T, Nair DG et al. Apoptosis induced by cryoinjury in human colorectal cancer cells is associated with mitochondrial dysfunction. Int J Cancer 2003; 103: 360–9.

21. Novick AC. Partial nephrectomy for renal cell carcinoma. Urol Clin North Am 1987; 14: 419–33.

22. Chosy SG, Nakada SY, Lee FT, Warner TF. Monitoring renal cryosurgery: predictors of tissue necrosis in swine. J Urol 1998; 159: 1370.

23. Woolley ML, Schulsinger DA, Durand DB et al. Effect of freezing parameters (freeze cycle and thaw process) on tissue destruction following renal cryoablation. J Endourol 2002; 16: 519–22.

24. Zlotta AR, Wildschutz T, Raviv G et al. Radiofrequency interstitial tumor ablation (RITA) is a possible new modality for treatment of renal cancer: ex vivo and in vivo experience. J Endourol 1997; 11: 251–8.

25. Schulman C, Zlotta A. Transurethral needle ablation of the prostate (TUNA): pathological, radiological and clinical study of a new office procedure for treatment of benign prostatic hyperplasia using low-level radiofrequency energy. Arch Esp Urol 1994; 47: 895.

26. Matlaga BR, Zagoria RJ, Woodruff RD et al. Phase II trial of radio frequency ablation of renal cancer: evaluation of the kill zone. J Urol 2002; 168: 2401–5

27. Farrell MA, Charboneau JW, Callstrom MR et al. Paranephric water instillation: a technique to prevent bowel injury during percutaneous renal radiofrequency ablation. AJR Am J Roentgenol 2003; 181: 1315–17.

28. McDougal WS, Gervais DA, McGovern FJ, Mueller PR. Long-term followup of patients with renal cell carcinoma treated with radio frequency ablation with curative intent. J Urol 2005; 174: 61–3.

29. Hafez KS, Novick AC, Campbell SC. Patterns of tumor recurrence and guidelines for followup after nephron sparing surgery for sporadic renal cell carcinoma. J Urol 1997; 157: 2067–70.

30. Bolte S, Ankem M, Moon T et al. MRI findings after laparoscopic renal cryoablation. Urology 2006; 27: 485–9.

31. Jang TL, Wang R, Kim SC et al. Histopathology of human renal tumors after laparoscopic renal cryosurgery. J Urol 2005; 173: 720–4.

32. Carvalhal EF, Gill IS, Meraney AM et al. Laparoscopic renal cryoablation: impact on renal function and blood pressure. Urology 2001; 58: 357–61.

33. Nadler RB, Kim SC, Rubenstein JN et al. Laparoscopic renal cryosurgery: the Northwestern experience. J Urol 2003; 170: 1121–5.

34. Johnson DB, Taylor GD, Lotan Y et al. The effects of radio frequency ablation on renal function and blood pressure. J Urol 2003; 170: 2234–6.

35. Gervais DA, McGovern FJ, Arellano RS et al. Renal cell carcinoma: clinical experience and technical success with radio-frequency ablation of 42 tumors. Radiology 2003; 226: 417–24.
36. Mayo-Smith WW, Dupuy DE, Parikh PM et al. Imaging-guided percutaneous radio-frequency ablation of solid renal masses: techniques and outcomes of 38 treatment sessions in 32 consecutive patients. AJR Am J Roentgenol 2003; 180: 1503–8.
37. Lee DI, McGinnis DE, Feld R, Strup SE. Retroperitoneal laparoscopic cryoablation of small renal tumors: intermediate results. Urology 2003; 61: 83–8.

12

Radiologic evaluation following renal cryoablation

W. Bruce Shingleton

Radiographic imaging • **Computed tomography** • **Magnetic resonance imaging** • **Conclusions**

It is estimated that 60% of renal masses currently detected are incidentially discovered.[1] The majority of these lesions are small and lend themselves to treatment by minimally invasive therapies such as cryoablation. While the technique of renal cryoablation is well understood, a critical portion of the assessment for this therapy is post-treatment evaluation.

There are two mechanisms which cause tumor destruction during the freeze process: direct cell injury and vascular injury. These occur as the result of the temperature in the tumor reaching $-20°$ to $-40°C$, which is the lethal temperature required for cell destruction. An important point to understand is that the leading edge of the ice front is $0°C$, which will result in only sublethal cellular injury. It is therefore necessary to extend the ice front 5–10mm beyond the tumor border in order that total cellular destruction occurs. The sublethal injury zone does appear as a hypervascular ring surrounding the cryolesion in some patients on post-cryo imaging studies.[2] This finding will be discussed in greater detail later in this chapter.

After a patient undergoes cryoablation for a renal tumor, the question arises as to how to best evaluate the response of the tumor to cryotherapy. Typically for a patient who undergoes a partial nephrectomy for a T1 tumor, current recommendations are for only a yearly chest X-ray and physical exam with no imaging of the kidneys.[3] Based on the results of 327 patients undergoing a partial nephrectomy at the Cleveland Clinic, it was noted that no patients with T1 disease had a local recurrence.[4] However, as cryoablation is a new minimally invasive treatment for renal tumors and long-term follow-up is not yet available, follow-up assessment of the ablated tumor needs to be performed.

What follow-up modality best assesses total tumor destruction? Some investigators have utilized percutaneous biopsy post cryosurgery for assessment of tumor destruction. Chen et al reported on 35 patients who underwent laparoscopic renal cryotherapy.[5] Twenty-one of the patients underwent CT-guided biopsies at 3 or 6 months post-cryo. All biopsies were negative for residual tumor and only demonstrated fibrosis and hemosiderin deposits. Nadler et al reported on 15 patients who had laparoscopic renal cryoablation performed.[6] Seven of 10 patients who had renal cell carcinoma underwent percutaneous biopsy 3 months post procedure with two of the seven biopsies positive for residual tumor.

Cestari and colleagues described their results in 35 patients who underwent laparoscopic renal cryosurgery.[7] CT-guided biopsies were performed in 25 patients at 6-month follow-up with all biopsies negative for neoplasm. From these studies, it appears that the vast majority of patients undergoing renal cryoablation have no evidence of residual tumor on repeat biopsy.

On the other hand, some studies have some difficulty in accuracy for renal tumor biopsies. One difficulty in reliance on post-cryo biopsies for determination of tumor ablation is the reported 16% false-negative rate for needle biopsy.[8] Dechet and collegues at the Mayo Clinic reported their study on prospective analysis of solid renal mass diagnosed with needle biopsy and the non-diagnostic rate was 20% and specificity only 60%.[9] Campbell et al described the results in 25 patients who underwent needle aspiration of renal masses with 25% of the biopsies being false negative.[10] Cestari reported one patient who had a negative post-cryo biopsy but subsequently had a suspicious lesion on follow-up MRI and was found to have renal carcinoma.[7] However, if a biopsy is obtained and demonstrates no viable tumor present, continuing radiographic follow-up is still necessary. If the cryolesion increases in size even in the presence of non-enhancement, repeat biopsy is warranted to rule-out recurrent tumor.

There has been no commonly accepted time interval to obtain post-ablation imaging studies. In early studies investigating cryoablation, MR scans were obtained on post-ablation day one.[11] Typically, these scans only showed hemorrhage with perfusion defects and were limited by post-procedure hemorrhage. There is no reason to obtain a post-procedure scan until a minimum of 1 month has lapsed to allow from resolution of any possible hemorrhage (Shingleton, unpublished work). Some investigators obtain the first scan at 3–6 months and if this scan demonstrates no enhancement, biannual scans are then obtained.[5,6,11] Our current recommendation is to obtain an imaging study at 1, 3, and 6 months. If the lesion is non-enhancing and stable in size, then biannual studies are obtained. In cases where the lesion has completely regressed, then annual scans are satisfactory.

RADIOGRAPHIC IMAGING

There are four imaging modalities available to evaluate tumor responses to cryoablation. These comprise ultrasonography, CT, MRI, and PET scans. At the present time PET technology is not sufficiently developed to the point of providing accurate assessment of tumor destruction after cryoablation and it is not recommended for routine surveillance imaging.

Ultrasonography is useful in documenting changes in linear size but is limited in its ability to assess the presence of viable tumor. There has been a recent report on the utilization of contrast-enhanced harmonic ultrasound for evaluation after cryoablation. Zhu et al described the ultrasound findings in three patients who had undergone renal cryoablation.[12] Using contrast-enhanced ultrasound, decreased enhancement was seen similar to that present on post-cryoablation CT scans. There was identified one case of persistent enhancement which was related to a local recurrence. Further evaluation in a larger series of patients would be required to determine the feasibility of this technique.

COMPUTED TOMOGRAPHY

CT imaging provides unique advantages over ultrasound in the evaluation of post-cryo tumors. The primary advantage is the opportunity to assess for the presence of

A
B

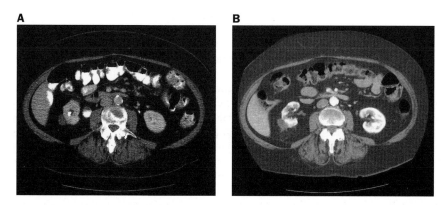

Figure 12.1 (A) Exophytic enhancing renal mass – pre-cryoablation. (B) Non-enhancement of renal mass – post-cryoablation.

viable tumor post-cryoablation. In order for this to be achieved, an unenhanced scan of the kidneys with thin 3-mm slices must be performed first. The administration of intravenous contrast is then administered and subsequent scanning undertaken. Typical radiographic appearance of the cryolesion is of non-enhancement. Figure 12.1 illustrates a renal tumor pre- and post-cryoablation on contrast-enhanced scans. It is an absolute requirement that no enhancement occur in the cryolesion. Any evidence of enhancement indicates there is residual tumor present and will require further treatment. In some circumstances, the cryolesion may have a larger diameter than the original tumor due to some hemorrhage secondary to probe insertion. Alternatively, the iceball may have been extended beyond the tumor border. This should not be a reason for concern as long as there is no enhancement present. Evidence of non-enhancement in the ablated tumor is the key requirement for evidence of tumor destruction. Rodriguez and associates reported their results of laparoscopic renal cryosurgery in seven patients in which contrast CT scans were performed at 3–6 month intervals and demonstrated perfusion defects at the ablated area with some tumor shrinkage.[13] Lee et al described their results in 20 patients after laparoscopic renal cryotherapy and at a mean follow-up of 14.2 months, no masses demonstrated residual enhancement in CT or MRI scans.[14] It has been documented that patients with residual enhancement in the cryolesion who subsequently undergo biopsy will be found to have residual disease.[15]

Another factor to be evaluated on post-cryo CT images is the size of the lesion. It has been documented that the tumor, post-ablation, will demonstrate a decrease in size as seen on scans as early as 3 months.[15] This most likely occurs as the result of a cellular response to cryoablation in which an acute neutrophil reaction begins with macrophage activity and absorption of cellular debris.[16] This leads to a decrease in size of the tumor along with fibrosis formation. Gill et al in their initial series of patients had 20% of their patients who had complete disappearance of the lesion.[11] Eleven of 15 tumors in Nadler's series decreased in size from 6 to 72 months in follow-up.[6] Shrinkage in tumor size can continue to occur over 6–12 months post-ablation. The key point is if there is any increase in size in follow-up period, the possibility of a tumor recurrence is present and a biopsy of the lesion recommended. This author

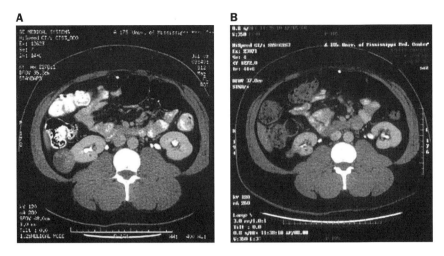

Figure 12.2   (A) Renal tumor pre-cryoablation. (B) Fibrotic remnant of tumor post-ablation at 1 year.

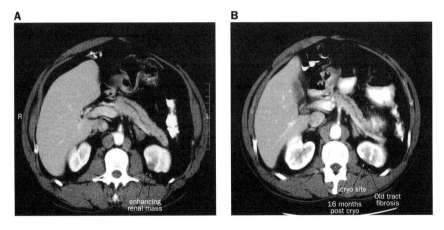

Figure 12.3   (A) Pre-cryoablation CT scan with parenchymal tumor. (B) Complete regression of tumor post-ablation at 16 months.

has treated one patient who had a non-enhancing but increasing-in-size lesion, and was found to have tumor recurrence.

Figure 12.2 illustrates the typical appearance of shrinkage in the tumor post-ablation with only a small amount of non-enhancing scar seen at 1-year follow-up. In some cases, the tumor will completely be reabsorbed and there will be no visualization seen on follow-up imaging, as seen in Figure 12.3. The case in Figure 12.3 additionally illustrates a common occurrence seen post-ablation, which is the presence of a small perinephric hemorrhage. These hemorrhages are typically seen in scans obtained early after the ablation procedure (1 day to 1 month). The hemorrhage can obscure

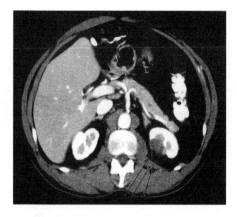

Figure 12.4   Residual enhancing renal tumor after cryoablation.

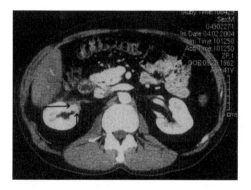

Figure 12.5   Recurrence of tumor 3 years after cryoablation.

clear visualization of the cryolesion; therefore, it may be necessary to repeat the scan in 1–2 months to be able to fully assess the cryolesion. It is important to note that if the cryolesion has increased in size over time, even without evidence of enhancement, the possibility of tumor recurrence may exist. At this point, biopsy of the lesion is recommended to rule out a recurrence.

The appearance of residual or recurrent tumor on CT imaging will be characterized by enhancement on post-contrast scans. Residual tumor can be noted typically on the first post-cryo scan obtained at 1 or 3 months. Figure 12.4 demonstrates the presence of a residual enhancing tumor after incomplete cryoablation. This image at 3-month follow-up showed the cryo defect created along with the residual enhancing tumor. Local recurrences can occur up to 3 years after ablation. Figure 12.5 shows a CT scan of a patient with a central recurrence 3 years after undergoing cryoablation. The enhancing portion of the tumor is clearly seen surrounded by the non-enhancing cryo defect. The pathologic examination found a 2.0-cm renal cell carcinoma surrounded by fibrotic scar tissue. It should be noted that there is a 4–18% incidence of multifocal disease in the ipsilateral treated kidney. In papillary adenocarcinoma, the

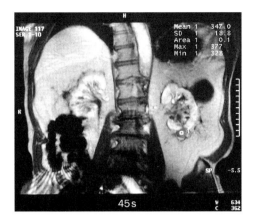

Figure 12.6   A peripheral rim enhancement sometimes seen on post-ablation MRI scans.

incidence of multifocality can be higher, underscoring the necessity for close radiographic follow-up.

MAGNETIC RESONANCE IMAGING

MRI has been utilized for post-cryo imaging by some investigators.[5,6] The use of MRI is mandated in some clinical settings such as patients with compromised renal function or contrast allergy for whom the use of contrast would be contradicted. If a patient has decreased kidney function, obtaining an unenhanced CT scan is unsatisfactory for the evaluation of tumor ablation. Remer et al described the MR imaging characteristics of cryolesions over time in 21 patients.[2] T_1, T_2, and T_1 gadolinium-enhanced images were obtained at day 1 post-cryo, 1, 3, 6, and 12 months after the procedure. On 1 and 3 months post-scan, the majority of T_1 images were isotense, and T_2 images were mainly hypointense and enhancement absent. Approximately 30% of lesions had a thin or thick rim of enhancement noted on T_1-enhanced images (Figure 12.6). The 6- and 12-month images showed T_1 images to be isotense, and T_2 images mainly hypo- or isotense, with no enhancement in T_1 gadolinium images. The peripheral rim enhancement which had been noted at 3 and 6 months had completely resolved at this time interval. As noted on the T_1-enhanced post-ablation image, the lesion had almost completely regressed in size. Remer noted that in 12 patients with 12-month follow-up, the cryolesion size decreased from 74 to 100% in size.[2] Additionally, perinephric changes were visualized in the scans at 1 and 3 months with increased signal intensity in T_2 images consistent with fluid accumulation. Lee and associates reported in their series of 20 patients treated with laparoscopic renal cryoablation, who were monitored post-ablation with CT or MRI.[14] Some patients had initial follow-up by CT then imaged with MR scans. No difficulty was noted in monitoring these lesions with these two modalities. Nadler reported that their patients were imaged with MR post-cryoablation in 13 of 15 patients.[6] All lesions were noted to be stable or decreasing in size with no enhancement.

Residual tumor after cryoablation will have a hyperintense signal on T_1 gadolinium scan. Figure 12.7 illustrates a cryolesion with peripheral enhancement on T_1 gadolinium image. Any evidence of enhancement in the region of the cryolesion, excluding a

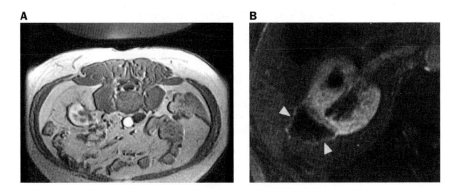

Figure 12.7   (A) T_1-weighted image post-gadolinium with exophytic lower pole tumor. (B) 7 month post-ablation T_1-weighted post-gadolinium image demonstrating peripheral enhancement (arrowheads). (Reprinted with permission of *American Journal of Roentgenology*.)

peripheral rim, should be considered viable tumor. From these investigators' experience along with ours, MR is a completely acceptable method of imaging cryolesions post-procedure. The difficulty that can occur is when follow-up MR scans are not performed at the same facility utilizing the same scanner. The software that is required for imaging varies according to the different capabilities of each MR unit. Therefore, there is no standard scanning technique used for MR imaging of the kidney.[17] If MR is utilized as the primary modality for monitoring of the post-cryolesion, it is important that the same unit and scanning technique be employed.

CONCLUSIONS

Renal cryoablation is an exciting advance in minimally invasive treatment of renal tumors. Radiographic follow-up is extremely important for the assessment of total tumor ablation and requires careful surveillance by the physician.

REFERENCES

1. Herts BR. Screening computerized tomography and the incidental renal mass. Urological implications of whole body scanning. AUA Update 2005; 24: Lesson 14.
2. Remer EM, Weinberg EJ, Oto A et al. MR imaging of the kidneys after laparoscopic cryoablation. AJR Am J Roentgenol 2000; 174: 635–40.
3. Janzen NK, Kim HL, Figlin RA, Belldegrun AS. Surveillance after radical or partial nephrectomy for localized renal cell carcinoma and management of recurrent disease. Urol Clin North Am 2003; 30: 843–52.
4. Hafez KS, Novick AC, Campbell SC. Patterns of tumor recurrence and guidelines for follow-up after nephron sparing surgery for sporadic renal cell carcinoma. J Urol 1997; 157: 2067–70.
5. Chen RN, Novick AC, Gill IS. Laparoscopic cryoablation of renal masses. Urol Clin North Am 2000; 27: 813–19.
6. Nadler RB, Kim SC, Rubenstein JN et al. Laparascopic renal cryosurgery: the Northwestern experience. J Urol 2003; 170: 1121–25.
7. Cestari A, Guazzoni G, dell'Acqua V et al. Laparoscopic cryoablation of solid renal masses: intermediate term followup. J Urol 2004; 172: 1267–70.

8. Zincke H, Dechet CB, Blute ML et al. Needle biopsy of solid renal mass. J Urol 1998; 159: 169A.
9. Dechet CB, Zincke H, Sebo TH et al. Prospective analysis of computerized tomography and needle biopsy with permanent sectioning to determine the nature of solid renal masses in adults. J Urol 2003; 169: 71–4.
10. Campbell SC, Novick AC, Hertz B et al. Prospective evaluation of fine needle aspiration of small, solid renal masses: accuracy and morbidity. Urology 1997; 50: 25–9.
11. Gill IS, Novick AC, Meraney AM et al. Laparoscopic renal cryoablation in 32 patients. Urology 2000; 56: 748–53.
12. Zhu Q, Shimizu T, Endo H et al. Assessment of renal cell carcinoma after cryoablation using contrast-enhanced gray scale ultrasound: a case series. Clin Imaging 2005; 29: 102–8.
13. Rodriguez R, Chan DY, Bishoff JT et al. Renal ablative cryosurgery in selected patients with peripheral renal masses. Urology 2000; 55: 25–9.
14. Lee DI, McGinnis DE, Feld R, Strup SE. Retroperitoneal laparoscopic cryoablation of small renal tumors: intermediate results. Urology 2003; 61: 83–8.
15. Gupta A, Allaf ME, Kavoussi LR et al. Computerized tomography guided percutaneous renal tumor cryoablation under conscious sedation: initial clinical experience. J Urol 2006; 175: 447–52.
16. Shingleton WB, Farabaugh P, Hughson M et al. Percutaneous cryoablation of porcine kidneys with magnetic resonance imaging monitoring. J Urol 2001; 166: 289–93.
17. Dunnich N, Sandler C, Amis E Jr et al. Textbook of Uroradiology, 2nd edn. 1997: 45–83.

13

Cryosurgery of adrenal tumors

Patrick Davol, John Danella

Introduction • Experience with adrenal-sparing surgery • Animal studies • Clinical studies • Technical aspects of adrenal cryoablation • Potential adrenal lesions amenable to cryosurgical ablation • Conclusions

INTRODUCTION

The use of cold temperature as a treatment of human tumors was first reported in 1851, when Arnott employed it to treat a uterine tumor.[1] Over the ensuing 150 years, cryosurgery has developed into a powerful treatment modality, utilized by various surgical and medical disciplines for the treatment of a multitude of different pathologic tissues. The advent of high-quality imaging modalities including computed tomography and high-resolution ultrasound has resulted in an increased detection of small intra-abdominal masses, and has further enhanced the ability of cryosurgery to deliver focal treatment to target tissues, offering an alternative to extirpative strategies for local cancer control and palliation of advanced disease. While cryosurgery is rapidly gaining acceptance in the urologic community for the treatment of prostate and kidney cancer, the cryosurgical experience with a variety of other urologic tissues is in it infancy.

The adrenal gland presents an excellent putative target for cryotherapeutic techniques, and may be uniquely suited to thermal ablative techniques for several reasons. First, adrenal tissue is susceptible to focal, controlled destruction by freezing, as evidenced by the results of animal studies. Secondly, conditions exist which make the adrenal gland susceptible to metachronous or bilateral disease presentation, increasing the importance of treatment modalities which can spare normal tissue. Thirdly, there already exists an extensive literature concerning laparoscopic approaches to the adrenal gland for extirpative and adrenal-sparing procedures, providing a clinical foundation for the exploration of alternative tissue-sparing techniques. Furthermore, early reports concerning the treatment of a variety of pathologic conditions of the adrenal gland with ablative techniques have begun to surface in the literature. This chapter will review the published literature concerning cryosurgery of the adrenal gland, and explore potential directions for future work.

EXPERIENCE WITH ADRENAL-SPARING SURGERY

The treatment of large or functional adrenal masses has evolved from open total adrenalectomy to laparoscopic adrenalectomy, with many centers now performing adrenal-sparing surgery. The argument for preserving normal adrenal tissue during extirpative surgery for adrenal masses has both a physiologic and pragmatic basis. While most patients retain adequate hormonal function, Nakada et al showed that patients treated for primary aldosteronoma with tumor enucleation retained a more robust hormonal response to angiotensin II and adrenocorticotropic infusion than those treated with total adrenalectomy.[2] Furthermore, this series showed no recurrence of hyperaldosteronism in either group at 5-year follow-up, providing a convincing rationale for the application of adrenal-sparing techniques in the treatment of functional adrenal tumors. Additional reasons to consider adrenal-sparing surgery include the dilemma facing patients presenting with bilateral disease, in which bilateral adrenalectomy results in the need for hormonal replacement and puts patients at risk for Addisonian crisis. While open partial adrenalectomy was described over 20 years ago, recent reports have described the technical feasibility and efficacy of laparoscopic adrenalectomy for adrenal adenoma, as well as pheochromocytoma.[3–6] The ability to spare normal adrenal tissue is of particular importance in patients with syndromes such as multiple endocrine neoplasia type 2 (MEN-2) and von Hippel–Lindau (VHL) disease, in whom it may be necessary to treat multiple, bilateral tumors either simultaneously or over time.

More recently, the use of radiofrequency ablation for the treatment of adrenal masses has been described. Wood et al performed image-guided percutaneous radiofrequency ablation (RFA) in eight patients. Both primary and metastatic lesions were treated. The authors found that 53% of lesions lost contrast enhancement and did not grow on follow-up imaging, while 20% had interval growth. They concluded that RFA was safe and well-tolerated, as well as efficacious in short-term follow-up, particularly for lesions < 5 cm in size.[7] With this background providing a practical and rational framework for the use of adrenal-sparing treatment modalities, a discussion of the developing role of cryoablation for treatment of adrenal masses is presented.

ANIMAL STUDIES

An important early study detailing the cryoablation of adrenal tissue *in situ* was reported in 1999 by Schulsinger and colleagues.[8] The authors studied the effects of both acute and chronic cryoablation in the dog using an open approach. A single 2-mm cryoprobe was placed 1 cm into the upper pole of the adrenal, and thermocouples placed both into adjacent adrenal tissue and the ipsilateral adrenal artery and vein. A single 15-minute freeze was conducted, with passive thaw until a temperature of 0°C was reached. A second group of dogs underwent laparoscopic adrenal cryoablation with a single 15-minute freeze cycle as in the open group, but were kept alive postoperative for 4 weeks before being euthanized. Histologic analysis of the adrenal tissue revealed clear areas of total tissue necrosis with adjacent viable tissue. The authors found that by 1 and 6 minutes of freezing, tissue-ablative temperatures were found at radii of 0.4 and 0.8 cm from the cryoprobe. They concluded that *in situ* cryoablation of adrenal tissue was safe, effective, and reproducible, and that even a single freeze–thaw cycle showed significant tissue destruction that did not lead to cellular regeneration at 4 weeks.

CLINICAL STUDIES

Following the work in the canine model, Munver and Sosa reported on an initial case of adrenal cryoablation in a patient with primary hyperaldosteronism and a 2.5-cm adrenal nodule. The investigators used a laparoscopic transabdominal approach to expose the adrenal, and placed a 3-mm cryoprobe into the nodule.

A single 15-minute freeze was completed, followed by passive thaw. The patient did experience a hypertensive crisis, which was controlled with IV antihypertensives. At 3-year follow-up, the patient's blood pressure was controlled with a 50% reduction in medication, and radiologic imaging had not shown an increase in the nodule size, although the authors did not describe whether there was scar present or any initial reduction in size.[9]

Cryoablation has also been used to treat metastatic lesions to the adrenal gland. Rohde and colleagues reported a case of cryoablation in the adrenal gland of a patient with metastatic renal cell carcinoma.[10] A percutaneous approach with MRI guidance was used to treat a 4-cm diameter lesion using an argon gas device with 2- and 3-mm cryoprobes. The tumor was treated with two 10-minute freeze–thaw cycles, and iceball extension carried at least 5 mm beyond the tumor margins. No complications were reported, and in follow-up imaging with CT at 6 months only necrotic tissue without enhancement was seen.

Other masses of the adrenal including angiomyolipoma (AML) have been treated with cryoablation (Rukstalis, personal communication), although experience is limited. No reports detailing the treatment of other tumors of the adrenal have as of yet been reported.

TECHNICAL ASPECTS OF ADRENAL CRYOABLATION

The technical details concerning the optimal approach for cryoablation of the adrenal gland have not been established. Open surgical approaches to the adrenal provide excellent tissue exposure and the ability to directly visualize iceball formation and monitor temperatures at the tumor periphery. While open cryosurgery of the adrenal has never been reported, much of the early work in renal cryotherapy was done via an open approach, yielding excellent early results.[11] However, in the current era of advanced imaging techniques and minimally invasive therapies, performing large open operations to deliver "minimally invasive" therapies seems counter-intuitive and a less-attractive option. Image-guided (CT or MRI) cryotherapy, while theoretically feasible, has not yet been described as a modality for primary adrenal pathology. However, using the already-established techniques employed for the percutaneous treatment of renal tumors, such an approach may be well-suited to the adrenal, particularly with the advent of 17-gauge cryoprobes which are easily placed percutaneously. Furthermore, the use of CT guidance for the treatment of adrenal lesions using radiofrequency ablation has already been reported, with at least two studies detailing the successful treatment of a small number of lesions in short-term follow-up, with few complications.[7,12] Limitations to this approach include the relatively small size of the adrenal gland and proximity to adjacent organs such as the spleen and liver, which may make percutaneous access with cryoprobes both difficult and potentially hazardous. Furthermore, the ability to treat larger lesions, which may necessitate the placement of multiple probes, could pose further difficulty with probe placement. Alternatively, laparoscopy affords excellent exposure to the adrenal, with the ability to directly visualize iceball formation, and as mentioned earlier has been successfully employed for adrenal cryoablation. The use of laparoscopic ultrasound, which in the authors' experience has been invaluable for the treatment of renal lesions, allows for accurate tumor localization and monitoring of the freezing edge during treatment. Both transperitoneal and retroperitoneal approaches are possible, and in the treatment of renal tumors both have shown similar efficacy and morbidity, although upper-pole and anterior lesions may be more easily accessed via a transperitoneal approach (Davol, unpublished data, 2005 AUA poster #1082).

Whatever approach is undertaken, adherence to the general principles of cryoablation as applied to the treatment of renal masses is advisable. The accurate placement of cryoprobes to ensure adequate tumor coverage during the freezing cycle is of the utmost importance, with multiple probes occasionally necessary if the treated lesion is >2–3 cm. The use of a double freeze–thaw cycle potentiates the cytotoxic properties of ice, especially in areas where the tissue may only just have reached lethal temperatures. The authors also routinely use temperature probes placed at the tumor periphery, as this is the only reliable means of assuring lethal temperatures in the areas of greatest importance, i.e. the tumor–normal tissue interface. Pretreatment biopsy and the use of tissue sealants may also be used depending on the clinical circumstances.

POTENTIAL ADRENAL LESIONS AMENABLE TO CRYOSURGICAL ABLATION

The multiple pathologic entities that may arise in the adrenal gland may all be potentially amenable to cryotherapy. As previously discussed, the published experience with adrenal-sparing surgery may serve as a foundation for the application of ablative strategies, and the few early reports detailing the use of radiofrequency add to this framework. Table 13.1 outlines the conditions which may be amenable to cryoablation. As previously described, cryosurgery has been employed for the treatment of functional adenomas, and this may prove to be its most important application. Multiple other lesions would theoretically be treatable as well, including angiomyolipoma and oncocytoma, lesions which have already been proven to be amenable to treatment in the kidney. The adrenal gland is a frequent site for metastatic lesions, and cryoablation may serve a useful palliative purpose in these instances. Interestingly, the lesion for whom this approach may be most problematic is pheochromocytoma. The consequences of freezing this lesion are unknown. It is possible that the insult afforded from cryoprobe placement and freezing may potentiate a hypertensive crisis either acutely or after the tumor thaws postoperatively, and it is unclear how effective standard antihypertensive medications would prove in this circumstance. It is also unknown how effective this approach would prove as opposed to standard surgical extirpation. If cryoablation of pheochromocytoma proves effective and safe, one could argue that this would be the preferred approach to the management of this condition, especially in the setting of MEN-2, in which bilateral disease is common.

Table 13.1   Adrenal conditions potentially amenable to cryoablation

1. Functional adenomas
   a. Estrogen- or adrogen-secreting cortical adenomas
   b. Aldosteronoma (Conn's syndrome)
   c. Cortisol-secreting adenomas
2. Oncocytoma
3. Angiomyolipoma
4. Adrenal metastases
5. Pheochromocytoma/MEN-2
6. Myolipoma

Clearly, further study is needed, and the availability of animal models may provide useful information before the technology is applied clinically.

CONCLUSIONS

Cryosurgery for the treatment of solid tumors is experiencing a renaissance. The adrenal gland offers an excellent putative target for this technology, and a limited but growing literature seems to indicate that cryosurgery will be an effective therapy for the treatment of a wide array of adrenal lesions. In particular, the ability to treat lesions in patients with syndromes predisposing them to recurrent, multiple, and/or bilateral tumors appears particularly valuable. As experience grows, and long-term follow-up data are reported, cryosurgery may well become the treatment of choice for the majority of adrenal lesions.

REFERENCES

1. Arnott J. On the Treatment of Cancer by Regulated Application of an Anesthetic Temperature. London: J Churchill, 1851.
2. Nakada T, Kubota Y, Sasagawa I et al. Therapeutic outcome of primary aldosteronism: adrenalectomy versus enucleation of aldosterone-producing adenoma. J Urol 1995; 153 (6): 1775–80.
3. Munver R, Del Pizzo JJ, Sosa RE. Adrenal-preserving minimally invasive surgery: the role of laparoscopic partial adrenalectomy, cryosurgery, and radiofrequency ablation of the adrenal gland. Curr Urol Rep 2003; 4 (1): 87–92.
4. Jeschke K, Janetschek G, Peschel R et al. Laparoscopic partial adrenalectomy in patients with aldosterone-producing adenomas: indications, technique, and results. Urology 2003; 61 (1): 69–72; discussion 72.
5. Walz MK, Peitgen K, Diesing D et al. Partial versus total adrenalectomy by the posterior retroperitoneoscopic approach: early and long-term results of 325 consecutive procedures in primary adrenal neoplasias. World J Surg 2004; 28 (12): 1323–9.
6. Walther MM, Herring J, Choyke PL, Linehan WM. Laparoscopic partial adrenalectomy in patients with hereditary forms of pheochromocytoma. J Urol 2000; 164 (1): 14–17.
7. Wood BJ, Abraham J, Hvizda JL et al. Radiofrequency ablation of adrenal tumors and adrenocortical carcinoma metastases. Cancer 2003; 97 (3): 554–60.
8. Schulsinger DA, Sosa RE, Perlmutter AA, Vaughan ED Jr. Acute and chronic interstitial cryotherapy of the adrenal gland as a treatment modality. J Endourol 1999; 13 (4): 299–303.
9. Munver R, Sosa RE. Cryosurgery of the adrenal gland. Technol Cancer Res Treat 2004; 3 (2): 181–5.
10. Rohde D, Albers C, Mahnken A, Tacke J. Regional thermoablation of local or metastatic renal cell carcinoma. Oncol Rep 2003; 10 (3): 753–7.
11. Rukstalis DB, Khorsandi M, Garcia FU et al. Clinical experience with open renal cryoablation. Urology 2001; 57 (1): 34–9.
12. Mayo-Smith WW, Dupuy DE. Adrenal neoplasms: CT-guided radiofrequency ablation – preliminary results. Radiology 2004; 231 (1): 225–30.

14

Economics of a cryoablation program

Michelle Nagel, Michael Enriquez, Daniel Hendricks

Financial and operational analysis • **Clinical applications** • **Case study** • **Proforma**
• **Summary**

FINANCIAL AND OPERATIONAL ANALYSIS

Background

Cryosurgery may be performed as an open surgical technique or as a closed procedure under laparoscopic or ultrasound guidance. The hypothesized advantages of
cryosurgery include improved local control and benefits common to any minimally
invasive procedure (e.g. preserving normal organ tissue, decreasing morbidity,
decreasing length of hospitalization). Potential complications of cryosurgery include
those caused by hypothermic damage to normal tissue adjacent to the tumor, structural
damage along the probe track, and secondary tumors, if cancerous cells are seeded
during probe removal.

Cryosurgery in the treatment of cancer began in the 1850s in London when breast
and cervical cancer were treated with iced saline solutions at a temperature of −18
to −22°C. The next advance, liquefaction of gases, occurred between 1870 and 1900.
Initial investigations involved non-urologic organs like brain, liver, skin, and rectum.
Renal cryosurgery began in the mid 1960s when kidneys were cooled with liquid
nitrogen in an effort to evaluate their functional recovery for purposes of transplantation. Subsequent investigations focused on the functional, morphological, histological, radiological, and technical aspects of renal cryoablation.

Description of the procedure

Cryosurgery or cryoablation is a technique involving the use of extremely low
temperatures to freeze and destroy tumors that are left in place to be reabsorbed.
It is a focal therapy that allows treatment of specific lesions with preservation
of normal tissue. Real-time ultrasound permits placement of probes and monitoring
of freezing since the developing iceball or cryolesion and the margin of normal
tissue frozen around the tumor can be seen. The freezing process involves insertion of hollow metallic probes through which liquid nitrogen circulates. The
probes are insulated except at the end of the shaft, which comes in contact with
the tumor.

Research has shown the procedure to be an effective and safe primary therapy for
localized cancer. The present challenge is for healthcare leaders to afford their patients
all available treatment options. Therefore, transferring the benefits of cryoablative

technology from large, academic medical centers to a rural hospital setting requires market evaluation and business savvy.

Resources

Cryoablation procedures can be performed in both freestanding outpatient surgery centers and inpatient facilities. All procedures are performed using a cryosurgical device with eight cryoprobe ports and an integrated temperature-monitoring system consisting of eight thermosensor sockets. The system relies on circulating argon and helium gases in its probes to freeze and thaw tissue, respectively. Varying the flow rate of argon gas to the individual probes regulates the freezing process. A biplane transrectal ultrasound probe is used to guide accurate probe placement and to monitor the freezing process. A computerized data system is used to continuously monitor and record all temperatures.[1]

CLINICAL APPLICATIONS

Cryosurgical ablation of the prostate (CSAP)

With the increase in the aging population and improved diagnosis, the incidence of prostate cancer has increased steadily over the past few decades. Approximately 200 000 new cases of prostate cancer were discovered during 2002, with greater than 70% of those cancers discovered while they are still localized.[1] Standard treatment options for localized prostate cancer include radical prostatectomy, external-beam radiotherapy, brachytherapy, and watchful waiting. With no clear optimal treatment option, novel therapies have developed over the past 20 years.

Cryoablation represents a novel treatment option that departs from the three established treatment options of modern prostate therapy: chemotherapy, radiation therapy, and surgery. As such, its acceptance and adoption as a primary treatment option by the urology community has been a slow process. Cryosurgery does offer advantages to other forms of treatment. The procedure itself takes approximately 2 hours to perform. Thus, patients either go home the day of surgery, or spend one night in hospital. Many patients resume normal daily activities in less than 1 week. Recovery is rapid and, unlike radiation, cryoablation can be repeated if prostate-confined cancer recurs. In fact, it is the only Medicare-approved treatment if localized cancer recurs after radiation therapy (brachytherapy or external beam).

Cryosurgical ablation of the prostate has been explored as a primary treatment alternative to surgery or radiotherapy for a select group of patients with clinically localized prostate cancer. It has also been explored as a second-line option for a select group of patients with residual or recurrent cancer following radical prostatectomy or irradiation. The proposed advantages of cryosurgical ablation are that the procedure is less invasive than surgery and recovery time is much shorter. The treatment involves the ultrasonic guidance of needles into the prostate through the perineal skin while the patient is under anesthesia. Liquid nitrogen is delivered to the prostate locally through each needle. The glandular tissue is rapidly frozen and thawed such that tissue necrosis follows. While external beam radiation therapy requires multiple treatments, typically only one treatment is required for cryoablation. Long-term statistics show that cryosurgery is at least as effective for low-risk cancers as radical prostatectomy and radiation. It has been shown to have better success rates than surgery and radiation for moderate- to high-risk cancers. It is Medicare-approved for both first-time and post-radiation occurrence.

Reimbursement

- The CPT code for this procedure is 55873 Cryosurgical Ablation of the Prostate (includes ultrasonic guidance for interstitial cryosurgical probe placement).
- The work relative value units (RVUs) for this procedure are 19.44.[2]
- The procedure has 90 postoperative global days.[2]
- Medicare covers cryosurgical ablation of the prostate as a *medically necessary* procedure only for the treatment of malignant neoplasm of the prostate. (ICD-9 diagnosis code 185 Malignant neoplasm of the prostate.[3])

Relative value unit (RVU) is the common scale by which practically all physician services are measured. The Centers for Medicare and Medicaid Services (CMS) and most other payors use RVU values to determine the reimbursement rate for services after incorporating geographic location and other factors. Practices may use RVUs to determine and measure productivity. All Medicare approved procedures have been given a Total RVU, which is a combination of three categories added together: Work RVU, Practice Expense RVU, and Malpractice Expense RVU. The *Work RVU* is determined based on the time it takes to complete the procedure and the difficulty level of the procedure. The *Practice Expense (PE)* RVU is based on the practice overhead and the *Malpractice Expense (ME)* RVU is based on the malpractice overhead of a given practice specialty. While the PE RVU and the ME RVU vary based on location and expenses, the Work RVU remains as a constant regardless of where the procedure is performed. The Work RVU is oftentimes used for benchmarking purposes in national productivity reports because it is a constant factor.

Global surgery is a standard package of preoperative, intraoperative, and postoperative services that are included in the payment for a surgical procedure.[4] Commonly referred to for the global days after a surgery has been performed.

Diagnosis code is a numerical classification descriptive of diseases, injuries, and causes of death: International Morbidity Code, Manual of the International Statistical Classification of Diseases, injuries and AMA Standard Nomenclature of Disease, etc.[4]

Medical necessity

Validating *medical necessity* is the key to successful healthcare procedure planning and reimbursement. When billing for Medicare services, the Centers for Medicare and Medicaid Services (formally HCFA) mandates that providers meet medical necessity guidelines according to their contractor's Local Coverage Determination Policies (LCDs) (formerly Local Medical Review Policies, LMRPs) and conform to many other coding conventions.

A decision made by appropriate professional staff after a service is provided as to the medical need for that service. The state-of-being thought to be required by the prevailing medical consensus. What is medically necessary in one period or one area may not be so in another.[4]

Medical necessity may also be defined as services or items reasonable and necessary for the diagnosis or treatment of illness or injury or to improve the functioning of a malformed body member.

CPT Assistant defines *medically necessary* services as those services or supplies that are:

- In accordance with standards of good medical practice;
- Consistent with the diagnosis; and
- The most appropriate level of care provided in the most appropriate setting.

Note that the definition of medical necessity may differ among insurers. Medically necessary services may or may not be covered services depending on the benefit plan.[5]

Revenue cycle operations management issues to consider

It is important to research what each individual payor determines as the appropriate process, documentation and necessary steps needed to ensure payment for each procedure performed (i.e. establishing medical necessity or having the appropriate referrals in place).

Payors or individual plans may only cover cryosurgical ablation of the prostate (CSAP) (55873) as a form of treatment for a prostate condition when preformed as the primary treatment for prostate cancer.

The local Medicare policy[3] for the case study area indicates that diagnosis code 185 must be documented and reported to support payment and Medicare medical necessity requirements.

- There must be clear documentation of the diagnosis contained within the medical record.
  - Coverage is provided for the use of CSAP, as a primary treatment for patients with clinically localized prostate cancer, stages T_1–T_3.
  - Salvage cryosurgery of the prostate for recurrent cancer is medically necessary and appropriate only for those patients with localized disease who:
    1. Have failed a trial of radiation therapy as their primary treatment, and
    2. Meet one of the following conditions:
       - Stage T_2B or below
       - Gleason score <9
       - PSA <8 ng/ml.
- Cryosurgery as salvage therapy is therefore not covered under Medicare after failure of other therapies as the primary treatment. **Cryosurgery as salvage is only covered after the failure of a trial of radiation therapy, under the conditions noted above.**

Professional reimbursement

- The professional charge for cryoablation of the prostate for the institution in the following case study was calculated to be $2655. When determining the appropriate charge for each institution it is critical to take factors into consideration such as: *payor mix and current payor contracts (percentage of charge vs. fee schedule)*.
- The range of professional reimbursement for this procedure varies from $936 to $1433 based on the payor and current contracts. The local Medicare carrier's professional reimbursement for this procedure is $1088.[2]

Hospital reimbursement

- The hospital facility charges may vary due to different lengths of time spent in the operating room or perioperative area and different supplies used on different patients, which would affect variable charges such as anesthesia or the recovery room time charge.

- If the procedure is completed in the operating room and the patient is admitted as an inpatient, the procedure will be paid based on a *diagnosis-related group (DRG)*.

Outpatient hospital reimbursement

- The average outpatient hospital facility charge used in this case study was calculated to be $22037.
- The outpatient hospital facility range of reimbursement varies from $770 to $12120 based on the payor and current contracts. The local Medicare APC payment for the institution studied in the case study is $6086. Medical Assistance (Medicaid) payment reimburses at a base rate for all outpatient charges.

Inpatient hospital reimbursement

- The inpatient hospital facility reimbursement is paid based on a Diagnosis-Related Group or DRG-based payment.
- Cryoablation of the prostate is categorized into DRG 334 Major Male Pelvic Procedure with co-morbidity *or* DRG 335 Major Male Pelvic Procedure without co-morbidity.
  - DRG 334: *Major Male Pelvic Procedures with cc.* The arithmetic mean length of stay (A/LOS) is 4.5 days. The average inpatient facility charge for DRG 334 was $37701. The ranges of inpatient facility reimbursement for DRG 334 vary between $7139 and $9465 for this case study. The Medicare reimbursement for DRG 334 is $9329.
  - DRG 335: *Major Male Pelvic Procedures without cc.* The arithmetic mean length of stay (A/LOS) is 2.9 days. The average inpatient facility charge for DRG 335 was $24336. The ranges of inpatient facility reimbursement for DRG 335 vary between $5284 and $7970 for this case study. The Medicare reimbursement for DRG 335 is $7104.

Diagnosis-related groups (DRGs)

System that reimburses healthcare providers fixed amounts for all care given in connection with standard diagnostic categories;[4] also defined as a classification scheme for grouping similar patients based on diagnosis, procedures and resource consumption.

Length of stay (LOS)

The length of an inpatient's stay in a hospital or other health facility. It is one measure of use of health facilities, reported as an average number of days spent in a facility per admission or discharge.[4]

55873 Cryosurgical Ablation of the Prostate			
	Average gross charges	Reimbursement ranges	Medicare reimbursement
Professional component	$2655	$936–1433	$1088
Outpatient facility	$22037	$770–12120	$6086
Inpatient facility DRG 334	$37701	$7139–9465	$9329
Inpatient facility DRG 335	$24336	$5284–7970	$7104

Cryosurgical ablation of renal mass

During renal cryoablation, the goal is to ablate the same amount of parenchyma that should be excised during an open surgical nephron-sparing procedure: the tumor itself and a surrounding margin of healthy parenchyma. A secondary healing process then occurs over time, with sloughing of the devitalized tissue and replacement of that area by a fibrotic scar. Certain aspects of cryosurgery are essential, including a rapid freezing, slow thawing, and a repetition of the freeze–thaw cycle. Rapid intracellular ice formation causes irreversible cell death. Lethal temperature for achieving reliable cell death is approximately −40°C. For normal and cancerous renal cells, a temperature of −20°C causes uniform necrosis.

Reimbursement

- The CPT code for this procedure is 50542 Laparoscopy, Surgical; Ablation of Renal Mass Lesion(s).
- The RVUs for this procedure are 19.97.[2]
- The procedure has 90 postoperative global days.[2]
- Reimbursement available for Renal Cryoablation only for the treatment of malignant neoplasm of the kidney (ICD-9 diagnosis code 189 Neoplasm, kidney, Malignant).
- Imaging Guidance can be reported separately from the surgical procedure as applicable. The applicable codes are:
  - **76940-26** Ultrasound guidance for monitoring tissue ablation
  - **76362-26** CT guidance for monitoring tissue ablation
  - **76394-26** MR guidance for monitoring tissue ablation.

Revenue cycle operations management issues to consider

It is important to research what each individual payor determines as the appropriate process, documentation, and necessary steps needed to ensure payment for each procedure performed (i.e. establishing medical necessity or having the appropriate referrals/authorizations in place).

- Individual payors may require a prior authorization for this procedure, in the best interest of ensuring payment; it is recommended that every planned cryoablation of renal mass lesion(s) be evaluated.
- Referrals may be required to be available and current prior to the patient visit.
- Payors or individual plans may only cover renal cryosurgery for select patients with small renal tumors less than 4 cm.

Professional reimbursement

- The professional charge for CPT code 50542 Laparoscopy, Surgical; Ablation of Renal Mass Lesion(s) for the institution in the following case study was calculated to be $6026. When determining the appropriate charge for each institution it is critical to take factors into consideration such as: *payor mix and current payor contracts (percentage of charge vs. fee schedule)*.
- The ranges of professional reimbursement for this procedure vary from $950 to $1265 based on the payor and current contracts. The local Medicare carrier's professional reimbursement for this procedure is $1081.[2]

Hospital reimbursement

- The hospital facility charges may vary due to different lengths of time spent in the operating room or perioperative area and different supplies used on different patients. This would also affect variable charges such as anesthesia or recovery room time charge.
- The average charge used was based on historical data when cryosurgical ablation of the renal mass lesion(s) was performed on the patient. All patient encounters found in the historical data included multiple procedures billed at the time of surgery, ultrasound guidance for monitoring tissue ablation (CPT 76940) and echography, retroperitoneal (CPT 76775).
- If the procedure is completed in the operating room and the patient is admitted as an inpatient the procedure will be a DRG usual payment.

Outpatient hospital reimbursement

- The average outpatient hospital facility charge used in this case study was calculated to be $26 350.
- The outpatient hospital facility ranges of reimbursement vary from $770 to $11 628 based on the payor and current contracts. The local Medicare APC payment for the institution studied in the case study is $2319. Medical Assistance (Medicaid) payment reimburses at a base rate for all outpatient charges.

Inpatient hospital reimbursement

- The inpatient hospital facility reimbursement is paid on a DRG-based payment.
- Cryosurgical ablation of the renal mass lesion(s) is categorized into DRG 303 Kidney, Ureter & Major Bladder Procedures for Neoplasm.
  - DRG 303: *Kidney, Ureter & Major Bladder Procedures for Neoplasm.* The arithmetic mean length of stay (A/LOS) is 7.7 days. The average inpatient facility charge for DRG 303 was $24 336. The ranges of inpatient facility reimbursement for DRG 303 vary between $11 400 and $15 170 for this case study. The Medicare reimbursement for DRG 303 is $15 170.

50542 Laparoscopy, Surgical; Ablation of Renal Mass Lesion(s)			
	Average gross charges	**Reimbursement ranges**	**Medicare reimbursement**
Professional component	$6026	$950–1265	$1081
Outpatient facility	$26350	$770–14492	$2319
Inpatient facility DRG 303	$24986	$11400–15170	$15170

CASE STUDY

The purpose of this section is to educate the reader regarding the financial impact of performing this procedure. The information present within this document is the scenario encountered by the facility studied and is dependent upon each institution's financial and reimbursement environment. The payor/patient population mix must be considered a variable in the analysis and subsequent conclusions drawn. This mix will have a substantial effect on the financial performance of this procedure.

Definitions

Listed are important terms that will be used throughout this section:

- *Actual Gross Charges*: the total charges of all utilization posted to a patient encounter. (professional & hospital).
- *Actual Net Revenue*: the revenue after contractual deductions based on payor contract.
- *Actual Variable Cost*: the actual variable cost of patient encounter (supplies, salaries, OR time, etc., to perform procedure).
- *Contribution Margin*: the net revenue less variable cost.

Environment

The system studied is a multispecialty system with 22 operating rooms. The OR cases studied were all performed in a hospital setting (no freestanding ambulatory cases). This hospital performed 17362 surgical cases, which would be considered large given the rural setting. This is a nationally recognized system that is a leader in advancing new technologies. The patient population consists of lifelong residents with little or no transient activity. For reimbursement purposes the Medicare classification for this facility is charge class 99, defined as all other Pennsylvania locations that are not classified as rural. Pennsylvania has two payment areas for physician services. They are charge classes 01 (Greater Philadelphia Area) and 99 (remainder of state). It is important to determine the local Medicare classification that applies to each individual facility.

Statistical data

The procedures reviewed were CPT 50542 Cryosurgical Ablation of Renal Mass and 55873 Cryosurgical Ablation of the Prostate. The analysis was performed on all cases (55) completed for a 10-month period since the inception of the procedure at this facility. The case mix was 23 inpatient cases and 32 outpatient cases. The payor mix varied as represented below:

Payor mix inpatient	43% – Medicare
	43% – Managed care
	14% – Commercial/fee-for-service
Payor mix outpatient	20% – Medicare
	67% – Managed care
	13% – Commercial/fee-for-service

Case data

The following represents a compilation of both prostate and renal cryosurgery data.

Per case	Inpatient	Outpatient
Gross charges	$31000	$26000
Net revenue	$13000	$7000
Variable costs	$9000	$10000
Contribution margin	$4000	($3000)

Case study conclusion

Cryoablation is most profitably performed as an inpatient procedure at this facility due to the increased hospital reimbursement captured within the payor mix. Based on the data provided, hospital reimbursement drives the profitability of this procedure because the CPT reimbursement would remain the same regardless of the patient status. Length of stay has a direct impact on the positive financial outcome. Top-notch facilities that focus on patient throughput can capitalize and create significant financial gains with this mindset. Note that the payor mix has a direct impact on the financial results due to the 24% increase in Managed Care outpatient versus inpatient. The hospital analyzed within this process has a substantial Managed Care population. Managed Care is not a suitable payor for the surgery inpatient or outpatient. It is profitable as an inpatient, but it is significantly lower than the other payors.

PROFORMA

Following are sample proformas providing a typical reimbursement and cost analysis for prostate and kidney cryosurgical ablation of tumors. In these proformas, the cryo-surgical procedural fees are based on the average fees provided by national companies that mobilize cryoablation equipment, supplies, and technicians to assist in performing cryosurgery. This analysis is intended to educate the reader on the financial breakdown of typical, uncomplicated cases. The Medicare reimbursement figures are based on general figures for the region in which the case study institution is located.

CRYOSURGICAL ABLATION OF THE PROSTATE
REIMBURSEMENT PROFORMA

MEDICARE INPATIENT

DRG 334-Major male pelvic procedure With complications or co-morbidity	$9,635

*Amount derived from 2005 CMS DRG Pricer
*Assume patients with less risk/complications
  would be performed as OP cases.

TYPICAL COSTS:

PROCEDURAL HOSPITAL COST: (OR Time $500, Recovery $250, Gas $300, Med/Surg Supplies $200, Pharmacy $100, Lab Chemistry $30; One (1) Inpatient Day @ $500)	($1,880)
Cryosurgical Procedure Fee Procedure Fee includes set-up, use of equipment, disposable supplies and technician (if applicable).	($5,000)
TYPICAL PROCEDURAL COSTS:	$6,880
HOSPITAL NET:	$2,755

CRYOSURGICAL ABLATION OF THE PROSTATE
REIMBURSEMENT PROFORMA

MEDICARE OUTPATIENT

APC CODE 0674 Payment (Locally Adjusted Rate 2005) $6,086
*APC calculation based on 2005 Proposed Wage Index
*Assume patients with less risk/complications
  would be performed as OP cases.

TYPICAL COSTS:

PROCEDURAL HOSPITAL COST: ($1,380)
(OR Time $500, Recovery $250, Gas $300, Med/Surg Supplies $200,
Pharmacy $100, Lab Chemistry $30) Supply list and cost outlined in
facility supply list

Cryosurgical Procedure Fee   ($5,000)
Procedure Fee includes set-up, use of equipment, disposable
supplies and technician (if applicable).

TYPICAL PROCEDURAL COSTS: ($6,380)

                                          HOSPITAL NET: (−$294)

CRYOSURGICAL ABLATION OF THE KIDNEY
REIMBURSEMENT PROFORMA

MEDICARE INPATIENT

DRG 303 Reimbursement $15,486
Kidney, Ureter and Major Bladder Procedures

*Amount derived from 2005 CMS DRG Pricer

TYPICAL COSTS:

PROCEDURAL HOSPITAL COST: ($3,280)
(OR Time $500 × 2 hrs., Recovery $250, Gas $300,
Med/Surg Supplies $500, Pharmacy $200, Lab Chemistry $30;
Assume Two (2) Inpatient Days @ $500)

Cryosurgical Procedure Fee   ($5,000)
Procedure Fee includes set-up, use of
equipment, disposable supplies and
technician (if applicable).

TYPICAL PROCEDURAL COSTS: ($8,280)

                                          HOSPITAL NET: $7,206

Average Supply Cost for Cryosurgical Ablation of Prostate

Argon Gas (1 tank 6000 psi)	**$225**
Helium Gas (1 tank 6000 psi)	**$75**
Miscellaneous Procedural / Disposable Supplies • Cysto Pack • Mayo cover • Basic IV (saline or water) bag 1000 cc (double spike) • .038 guidewire • Suprapubic catheter kit • Foley catheter 22 Fr • Toomey syringe 60cc • 4 × 4 gauze • Prep Kit • KY Jelly • Saline 1 Liter bottle × 2 • Condom for Ultrasound Probe • Sterile Towel Pack • Surgical Gown • Sterile Gloves	**$200**
OR Time (1 hour) Typical Staff: 1 – Scrub & 1 – charge nurse	**$500**
Recovery Time (1 hour)	**$250**
Laboratory Chemistry (Hematocrit, Basic Metabolic Panel)	**$30**
Pharmacy Drugs: Typical Drugs administered during stay include: Ephedrine Sulfate, Pavulon Inj, Sodium Chloride Inj., Xylocaine Inj 2%, Kefzol 1 gm, Glycopyrrolate 1 mg, Succinylcholine 200, Lidocaine Inj 1%, Thiopental Inj 500 mg, Sublimaze, Versed)	**$100**
Total Supply Cost	**$1380**

Argon and Helium Gas Specifications

Argon
Grade 5 / 99.9% pure
Tank Size: 10″ Diameter × 51″ Height
6000 psi High Pressure
Weight: 360 lbs
Regulator: CGA 677

Helium
Ultra High Purity Grade
Tank Size: 9″ Diameter × 55″ Height
Pressure @ 6000 psi (standard size)
Weight: 150 lbs
Regulator: CGA 580

Note: Vendor provides regulators for tanks.
Note: Your normal distributor should have the Helium in stock, but the Argon will be a special order due to the high-pressure requirements.

SUMMARY

Choosing the appropriate treatment option for prostate cancer can be complex. Scientific and technological advances over the past decade have challenged the established diagnostic treatment paradigms regarding prostatic adenocarcinoma. Cryoablation represents a novel treatment option that departs from established treatment options of modern prostate therapy. As such, its acceptance and adoption as a primary treatment option by the urology community has been a slow process. Cryosurgery does offer advantages to other forms of treatment. It is a minimally invasive technique with low morbidity. Thus, patients are released home the day of surgery, or spend one night in hospital for routine observation. Many patients resume normal daily activities in several days. Recovery is rapid, and unlike radiation, cryoablation is a repeatable treatment if prostate-confined cancer recurs.

Developing a viable and stable cryoablation program is dependent upon patient selection, access to technology, physician education, and financial viability. This is accomplished through key physician partnerships to utilize current technology and proctor physician education. While capital resources are often more accessible in large teaching institutions, the goal of physician and healthcare leaders should be to provide the spectrum of treatment options to all patients. Patient selection in treatment personalizes their care and reinforces compliance. The health system used in the preceding case study is focusing administrative efforts to establish a mechanism to mobilize this technology for use in regional hospitals. Key to these efforts is the collaborative relationships developed between physicians in the region. Physicians skilled in cryoablation will proctor local urologists. This type of technology-mobilization company will be modeled after the joint venture model used by mobile lithotripsy companies. The venture strategy is to educate proctor physicians on the latest technology and interventions in cryoablation and make available the necessary resources (equipment) to provide these services. The goal will be to educate these physicians on new interventions and technology and work with their affiliated hospitals to bring resources for their use.

Program strength is also dependent upon financial stability. Each organization will need to assess its third-party contracts and adjust its model accordingly. The disparity between outpatient and inpatient reimbursement presents stiff challenges. Industry leaders, physicians, and patient advocacy groups have lobbied CMS to reconsider proposed decreases in outpatient payments for cryoablation. Data indicate that this procedure is well tolerated in an outpatient setting for both patients and physicians. Hospitals of all sizes are presented with the pressure to provide state-of-the-art interventions for their patients while maintaining the financial foundation of their institution.

REFERENCES

1.   Ellis DS. Cryosurgery as primary treatment for localized prostate cancer: a community hospital experience. Urology 2002; 60 (2A): 34–9.
2.   2005 Medicare Physician's Fee Schedule (Pennsylvania Charge Class 99).
3.   HGSA/CMS Policy S-108F Cryosurgical Ablation of the Prostate (CSAP).
4.   Medicare Part B Reference Manual, Appendix A, Glossary of Medicare Terminology.
5.   CPT Assistant, Summer 1992, page 21.

Index

prostate-specific antigen (PSA)
  as disease control surrogate endpoint
    43, 44
  tumor assessment after cryoablation
    35, 36
prostate tumors
  pathologic findings after 34
  persistence after cryotherapy 9, *34*,
    34, *Plate 2*
  ProstaScint scans *26*, 26
PSA *see* prostate-specific antigen (PSA)
PSA bounce 47
PSA doubling time (PSADT) 47
PSA failure
  algorithm for *52*
  see also biochemical recurrence
PSA nadir 47

quality of life
  assessment tools 67
    EORTC instrument 69
    FACT-general form 68
    FACT-P 67–9, *69*
    Sexuality Follow-Up Questionnaire
      68
  after brachytherapy 68
  after external beam radiotherapy
    68–9
  after prostate cryosurgery 67–70
  after radical prostatectomy 69

racemase 35, *36, Plate 3*
radical prostatectomy 69
radiofrequency ablation
  for adrenal masses 138
  approaches/access 121–2
  background 120
  complications 124–5
  follow-up 122–3
  indications 118
  kill zone estimation 120
  probes 120
  and renal function 123–4
  systems available *121*
  technique 120–1
  vs cryoablation 117–37
  vs cryoablation
    access 121–2
    complications 124–5
    outcomes 122–4
    percutaneous renal 105
radiologic evaluation after renal
  cryoablation 129–36
  computed tomography 130–4

magnetic resonance imaging 134–5
  ultrasound 130
radiotherapy
  adjunctive 10, 97
  failed
    evaluation of local recurrence 47–8
    radio-recurrent prostate cancer 48
    salvage cryotherapy after 34–5
  vs cryotherapy 117–27
recrystallization 6
recurrence *see under specific
    conditions/procedures*
reimbursement
  prostate cryoablation 145
    hospital 146–7
      inpatient 147
      outpatient 147
    professional 146, 147
  renal cryoablation 148–9
    hospital
      inpatient 148
      outpatient 148
    professional 148
renal ablation 117–37
  algorithm for *118*
  approach 117–18
  background 117
  cryoablation *vs* radiotherapy 117–27
  follow-up 122–3
  indications/contraindications 117
  natural history, post-ablation 122
renal cell carcinoma 85
  cells surviving cryotherapy 86
  persistent 91
  size of lesions detectable 85
renal collecting system
  experimental cryoablation 104
  radiofrequency ablation injuries 124
  resistance to cryogenic injury 72, 87,
    114, 124
renal cryoablation 148–9
  advantages/disadvantages 75, 88–9
  approaches/access 121–2
  background 118
  clinical outcomes 85–101
  clinical series *91*
  complications 94, 96–7, 124–5
    frequency *95*
  contraindications 88
  cryobiology 71–2, 86–7
  cryoinjury and urinary extravasion
    86
  deviations from optimal technique 9
  effects on tissues 86, 103–4